Half the Man I Was With Twice the Heart
The Danny Coleman Story

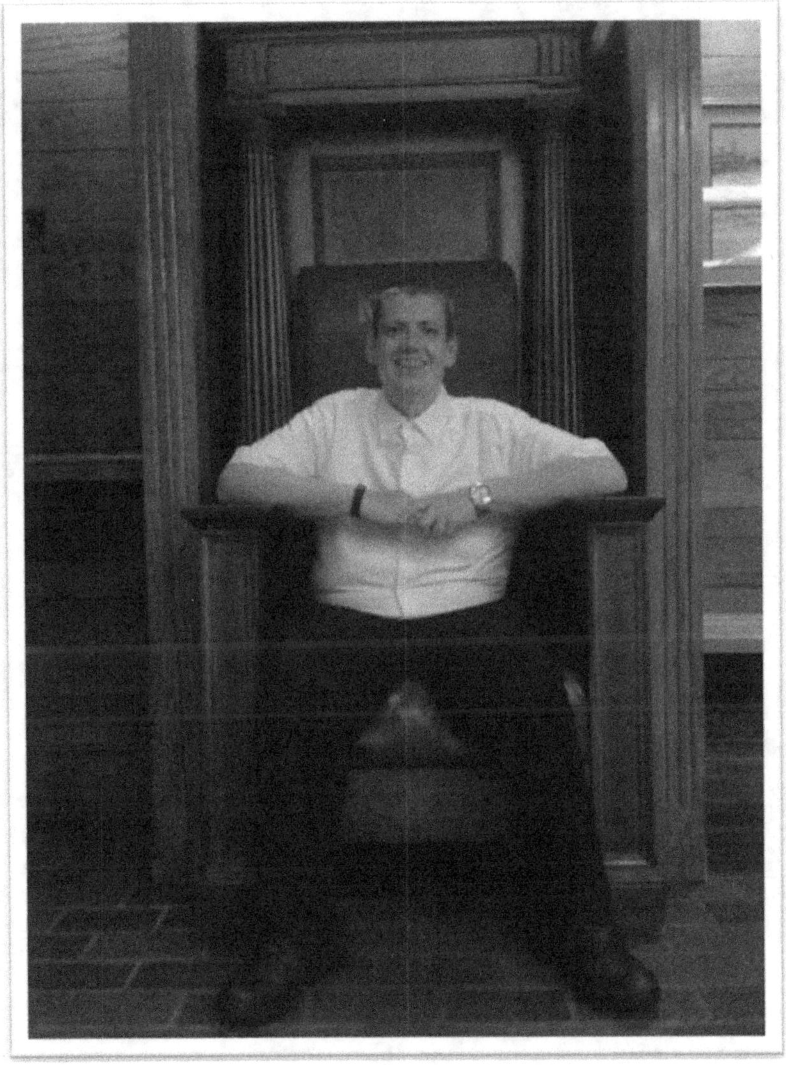

Told to and Written by
Kathleen Mary Capossela

Half the Man I Was
With Twice the Heart
The Danny Coleman Story

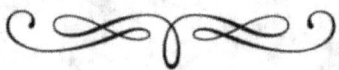

Told to and Written by
Kathleen Mary Capossela

Contents

Forward

By Ben Braswell

Philippians 4:13: I can do all things through Christ which strengtheneth me.

I met Danny when we were playing baseball for a Dixie Youth team. We were fast friends and we shared a love for America's pastime, baseball.

We reconnected several years later and soon, we began to talk daily. Danny struggled with his weight, but never with his heart.

Though we would trade ball cards, our real bond was formed through a purpose.

Danny attended a center and soon shared with me a secret. He had a mental health issue. I didn't know what this was, as Danny was just a good ole boy. However, as our friendship developed so did our conversations.

Danny shared with me his purpose. He loved people and wanted to share the gospel of Jesus with them. Though Danny had a big heart, he had major obstacles-- his weight and his mental health. It was very tough to see him go through the challenges the weight brought as well as some mental breakdowns along the way.

In the bible, God continually used those who seemed unworthy such as a tax collector, a fisherman, and so on. Thank God he doesn't call the qualified, but calls the willing. In many a conversations he and I would talk about God's plan for our lives. Despite his obstacles, Danny never seemed down. Don't get me wrong, he struggled with major depression, but he was more worried about me.

The truth is, he's ordained with an anointing and I'm glad to call him my brother in Christ and my friend. His selflessness, dedication, and determination sum up who he is.

Many people go their whole lives not knowing their purpose. This saddens me to think that there are people, maybe even reading this book, who don't know their purpose. If there is anything that Danny knows, it's that God put him on this earth to struggle, then overcome so that others would know that anything, I mean anything, is possible with God.

I hope anyone who reads this book is blessed to know about the journey that Danny has taken. I pray that those who read this book know Jesus is the answer to your problems and he will deliver you if you trust Him. I was humbled to witness Danny's journey first hand. Even Though he is "half the man" he used to be, he has twice the heart as most.

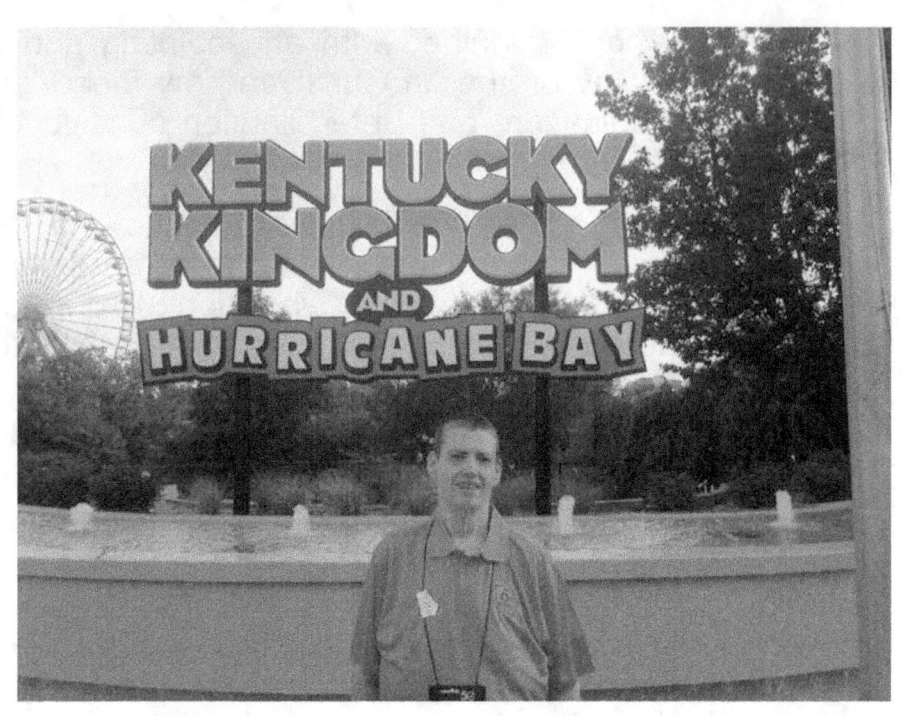

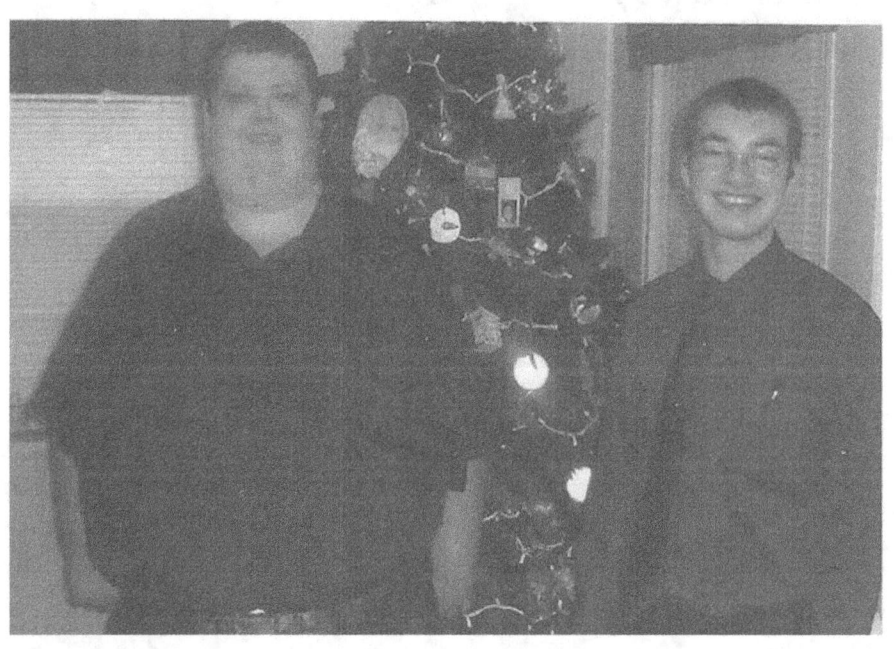

Dedication

I would like to dedicate this book to my wonderful Grandmothers. My Grandmother Nancy Coleman better known to me as Mink, was a constant companion to me in my early years until I was about 16 years old when she passed away of Cancer. I have many fond memories of time spent with my Grandmother Mink. The times when she would be there to cheer me up when times were tough. She always loved to fix me my favorite foods and offered me great comfort when I was having trouble in life. My Grandmother Mink was taken away from me when I was 16 years old so she never got to see me graduate from High School or College, and she never got to see me take control of my life and my health and stopped my march down the road to a premature death. However I know she is in Heaven looking down on me watching over me and I know she is proud of the man I have become.

I want to dedicate this book to my Grandmothers because they have always been there for me when I needed them. Through my story and the mark I leave upon this planet, may the memories of my Grandmother Mink live on with me. She was a very kind, humble, Christian lady and I am eternally grateful for the time God allowed me to spend with her here on Earth.

I also cannot leave out my Grandmother Molly. She is equally important to me and I don't know what I would do without her. She has always been super supportive of my endeavors to take back control of my health.

She was also there to help support me through one of the roughest times in my life when I suffered from a debilitating Mental Health diagnosis. Family is a very important part of my life and I have many fond memories of family gatherings at Grandma Molly's house for different holidays including Easter, Thanksgiving, and Christmas. And when my family has a get together we don't have food we have a feast which is a blessing and a curse. I would not be the man I am today if it were not for the love and support and compassion from both my Grandmother Mink and my Grandmother Molly. I am eternally grateful for God placing both of these ladies in my life. I could not have picked a better family if I were given the option to choose my family.

Grandmother Mink I will always love and miss you but I can rest knowing that you are in Heaven with our Lord and Savior Jesus Christ and I will see you again someday. Grandmother Molly I also will always love you and am thankful for all you have done for me through the years. I wish I could do for you a small portion of what you have done for me in a large way. I love both of you and may God bless you!

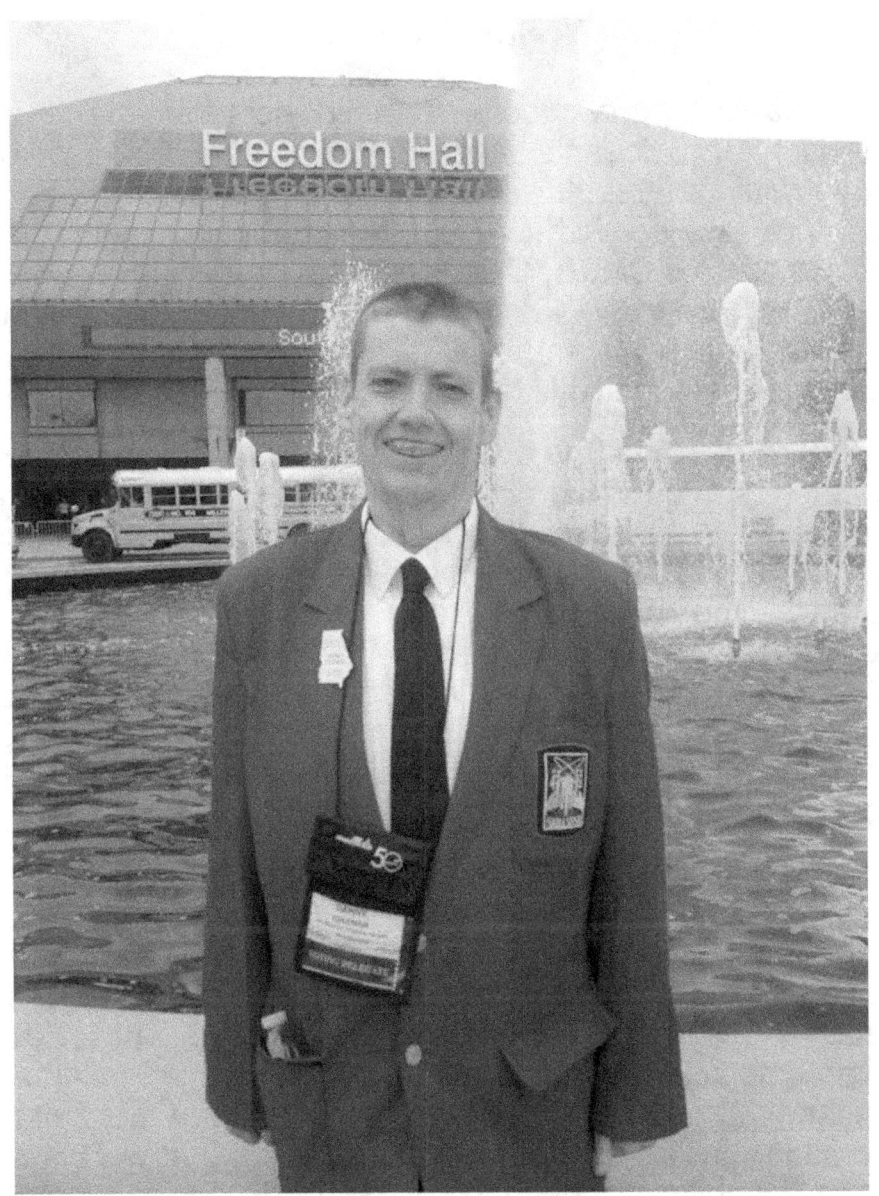

Introduction

It starts in preschool. A child acts out, can't pay attention and doesn't seem to be able to focus or get along with others. In time they are evaluated and soon they are labeled with particular alphabetical tags: ADD, ADHD, CAPD, CARS, DD, and TS to name a few. Pretty soon they are treated differently, and when other children want to know what the deal is, the explanation is simple that the labeled child is 'special'.

As life goes on, the special child may have episodes of happiness and function in wonderfully normal ways but as time passes, the differences that make the child special can create some painful complications: pointing fingers, name calling, bullying. At one point the names change from ugly, funny and stupid to crazy, nut job and psychopath. The name calling doesn't stop at high school or graduation; it can often seep into the lives of simple ordinary adults who have but one desire in mind, to be accepted and treated with dignity.

Mental Illness affects 26.2 percent of Americans ages 18 and older. One in every four adults suffers from a diagnosable mental disorder in a given year. This translates into a walloping 57.7 million people in our nation. Many of those afflicted can control their symptoms with the help of counseling and medication and live healthy happy lives, but in many parts of our culture, the name calling continues and the labels that were set in place as children continue to dangle from the necks of those affected well into adulthood.

I know what it's like to suffer from a mental illness. I struggled throughout my childhood and into my teens with fears and paranoia, but I knew what it was like to be different, to have one of those labels; I knew what it was like to be ridiculed, talked about, made fun of and called names. I was determined to be normal, I fought the stigma of being the crazy one throughout my young years and I was determined to not allow anyone to see a weakness in me that would in any way lead to the conclusion that I was 'special'.

I had a good family--they loved and supported me through my school years and into adulthood.

I managed to convince everyone that there was nothing different about me--I was fine, normal with a capital N, and in no way did I allow them to tease me or make me out to be the oddball or the one off my rocker.

But that all changed when I was 23 years old, I can't really explain how it all started, things began to shift in my head and I started to feel peculiar. My fears were out of control and at one point I had difficulty trusting people and leaving my house without entering into a serious panic attack. I was afraid all of the time, and the fact that I was very overweight did not help or make me feel any better. I needed help, that was certain, but I didn't ask for help because I didn't want to be called crazy, so I held on to my sanity and tried to make the best of it. Until one day I lost it and fell victim to a disease that was in no way my fault.

Having a breakdown landed me in a mental hospital and that was the beginning of my education. I saw mental illness first hand, and it devastated me. At one point in my recovery I was afraid to deal with the doctors and the medication because I thought if I would just pretend everything was okay if I could just act normal and ignore my symptoms, I could convince my family and all of my doctors that I was good, normal like everybody else.

But you cannot ignore mental illness, it's not like a cold: take vitamin C, drink lots of juices and in a couple of days you're all fine and good. It does not go away simply because you will it to, it has to be dealt with.

Once you do, facing the reality of your situation and submitting to the care of a good psychiatrist can mean the difference between running scared, lying awake all night praying it will get better and actually getting better, seeing your condition improve and interacting in life's daily issues with joy and normalcy.

Being diagnosed with a mental illness is not the end of the world, and people should not treat you as such. All human beings have imperfections and frailties--what doesn't break us, makes us stronger. Dealing with a mental illness can be complicated, but it is very possible to live happily, to be successful and have the confidence of knowing that you are in charge of your life and fully capable of a life of dignity.

I've made it a big part of my life to create mental health awareness, to educate people, to show them that in no way does the person suffering from a mental illness whether it be bipolar disorder, Asperger's Syndrome, borderline personality disorder or schizophrenia, once properly diagnosed and properly treated, people with a mental health disorder can move on in life and discover all of its joys and wonders with no drawbacks and most assuredly, without being labeled as special or different.

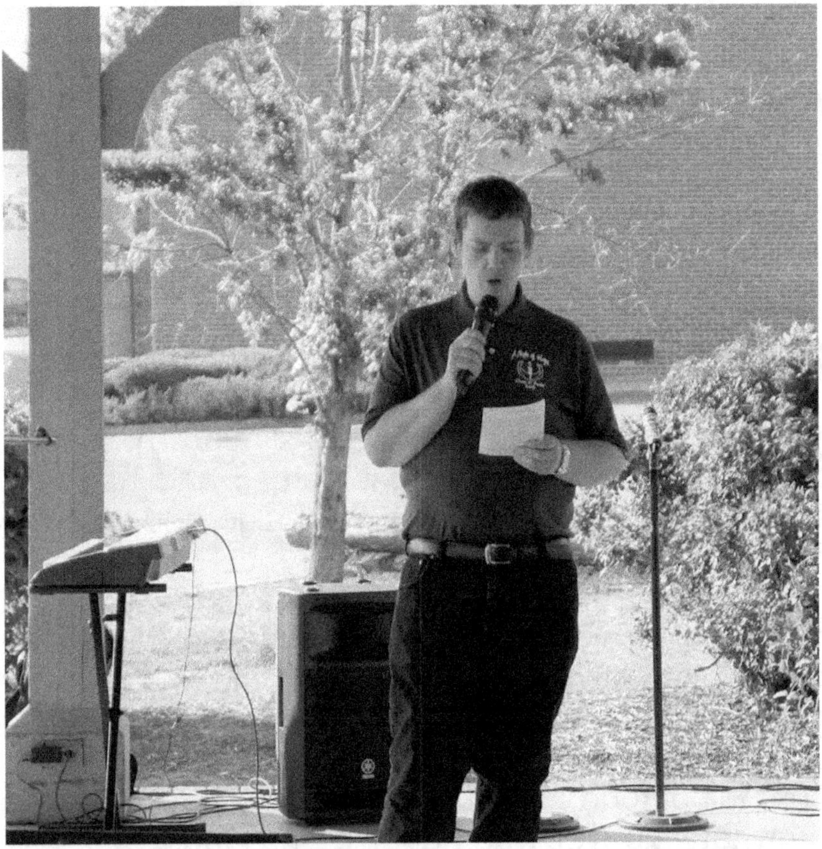

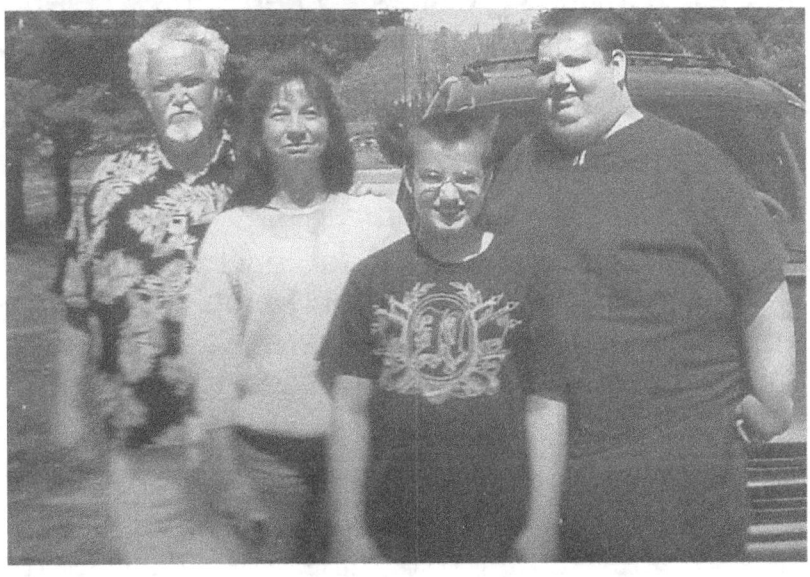

Chapter 1 - A Simple Life

I was born and raised in a small town in South Georgia. My father was a truck driver and not afraid of hard work. He was a big man and while I will say his size hurt him in some ways, he never let it keep him from doing the important things and he was a good dad and a wonderful provider.

My mother was a gentle woman, very disciplined in the matters of diet and always tried to be supportive of me when I would try to lose weight and slim down. She had a problem with being overweight herself and had learned from experience how to battle the bulge and when I was partaking in that battle, she was most supportive and encouraging. There was a big obstacle for me with my family when it came to trying to maintain a healthy eating plan. We were always having a gathering to celebrate one thing or another; birthdays, anniversaries, holidays. It didn't matter what it was, we were ready to celebrate with a room full of food and hungry people. It got to where we knew what whoever was bringing and would look forward to those particular dishes when the celebrating commenced. It all took place at my Grandma Molly's house and there was no denying it, there was enough food to feed an army, but we didn't let that stop us from going full force into the casseroles, meats, and desserts set before us.

There were tables set up for each particular item. Desserts were plentiful and the only problem I discovered was the size of the plates. There was just none big enough to provide the space needed to hold all of the food I wanted.

There was so much food being passed around, it was hard for one to decide on what was a favorite, but I pretty much discovered that I had mine. My Aunt Geraldine made this delicious macaroni and spam casserole that I was ready to dig into as soon as we were given the signal to eat. There was always a special plate of deviled eggs made by my sweet Grandma Molly set aside with my name on it. I remember the joy I experienced every time I saw that plate of eggs stuffed with delicious perfection made by my sweet grandma.

With so much celebrating going on, I was beginning to lose belts, I ran out of holes a few times and soon I was moving into new pants. I gained a few pounds in my childhood and by the time I got into my teen years, I experienced the pain of being made fun of and the torment of being picked on by others who called me names and made me feel bad. I soon discovered that I had to work hard to keep myself on the edge of 'not too fat' and when those celebrations hit, it was all I could do to keep from losing it and going overboard with gluttony.

My mother taught me that the way to lose weight and keep it off was with eating salads and walking a lot every day. I didn't mind the salads now and again and I tried to stay active, but when my mama made her specialty, what she called Chinese Pudding, I sort of lost the health and fitness incentive and gave into the mashed potatoes, ground beef, gravy and generous amounts of peas and corn.

For the most part, I held strong trying to stay healthy and as slim as I could, but eventually I gave into the boredom that sometimes filled my life and I was often driven to my favorite junk foods. I don't know what it was about the salty, crispness of potato chips, but there were times when I felt bored to the point of tears and the only thing that could cheer me up was a bag of my favorite chips.

Now and again I was driven to the television for company and I always enjoyed watching my favorite shows, but I soon learned that it was so much more enjoyable sitting down to a television show with my friend Reese, you know the guy who made those peanut butter cups? I could eat a lot of those little cups and enjoyed them immensely.

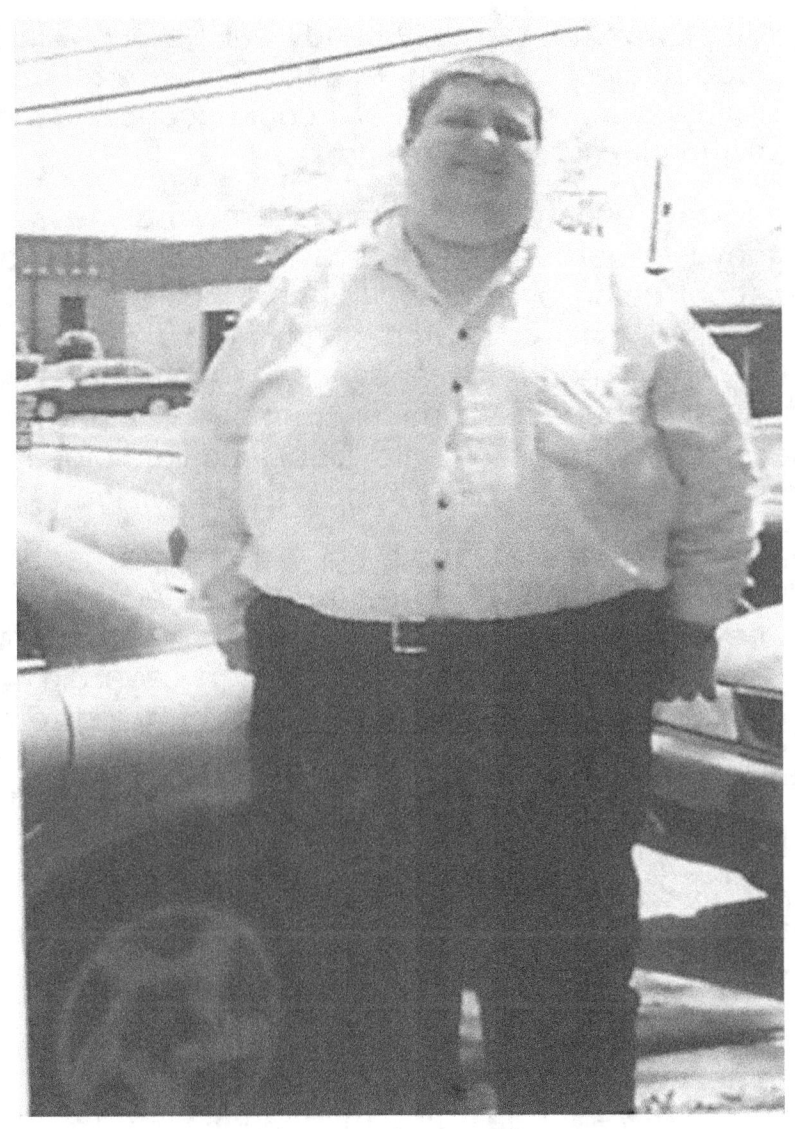

But that was not the only candy bar I brought into my entourage against boredom, I soon discovered that there were many sweet morsels that I could count on to make me feel the pleasure of snacking.

I had my favorites and I made it my business to be sure they were around when I was feeling bad and out of sorts about being by myself. When I look back to those days when I was in search of just the right goody to encase in my need for a snack, I can't forget those delightful little bundles of cake wrapped in goodness that came in the form of a Little Debbie cake, those were always good for a day off in front of the television.

Back then I was a simple kid with simple needs and food was not ineludibly a threat--it was a necessary thing and I never felt like I had a problem with it. I thought this was normal, the thing that everybody my age did; when we got together there was always talk of going to get a pizza or some ice cream, so food was just the same way, they could eat an entire pizza and never seemed to gain a pound.

This was one of those things that I thought was so unfair, something that everybody used to be social, like me and my family with our gatherings.

But I soon learned that food did not affect everybody the same way. I wanted to know why I was having a problem with weight gain and my friends were not. I was always a heavy kid, I was always teased for it, but it didn't seem fair to me that I would eat just as much as the kids in my family and they never seemed to get fat. I have some cousins who put a hole in a table full of food, suck down a gallon of sweet sodas and hit the dessert tables five or six times before they were ready for a nap and they never seemed to gain a pound. Me, on the other hand, it seemed like all I had to do was look at the food and it put a strain on my belt. I had friends who were so cruel in my younger years. I tried to be okay about it, I tried to understand the reality of genetics and not everybody being the same and just accepting my fate but I could never really understand what was happening in my body and what made me so different from everybody else?

There were times when I would feel absolutely embarrassed by eating foods, thinking that everybody saw me as the fat kid who just couldn't get enough. This led me to be a bit fearful of what others were thinking about me and I soon became a little paranoid about what others were thinking of me. In time I felt the strain of being the fat kid and I wanted to change that but no matter how hard I tried, I could never escape him.

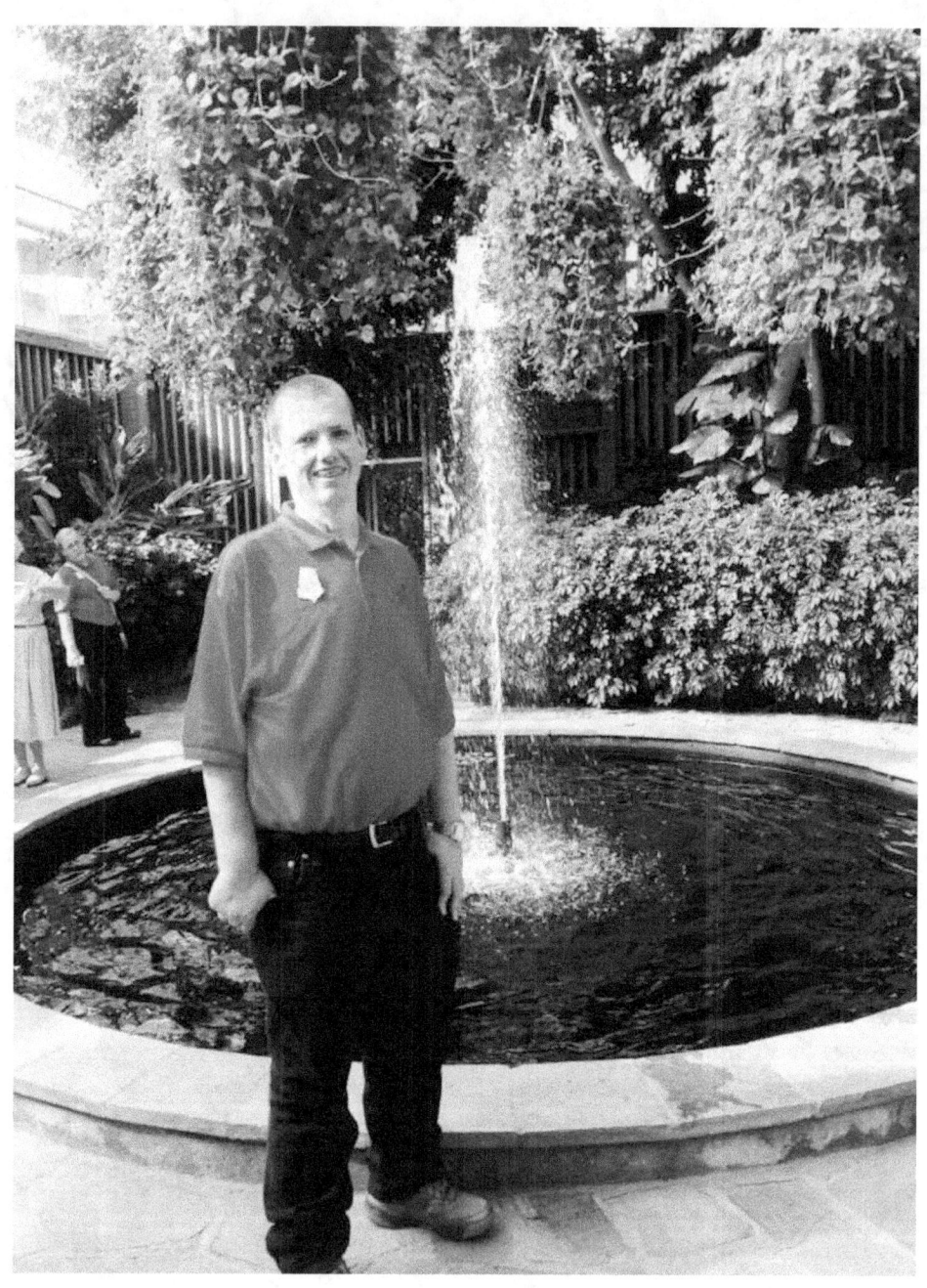

Chapter 2 - Finding Comfort

We all have special people in our lives, people who love us in a particular way who have the power to make us feel good even on our worst day. I was blessed to have a good family who loved and supported me no matter what and I will always be grateful for that.

One of the most wonderful people who I look back on fondly with great respect and appreciation is my grandmother, I called her Grandma Mink. I'm not really familiar with how that nick name came about, I just know that when I spoke to her this is what I called her and today when I recall the angel from my past who always made me smile and took me from a frown to a smile it was my Grandma Mink.

Grandma Mink was very much in love with her husband, Olvie. They had an undying devotion for each other. They spent a lot of time together and depended on one another.

When my grandfather passed away, my grandmother was heartbroken and fell into a state of despair. She thought that her life was over. She thought that she was ready to leave the earth and saw nothing here for her. Until November 7, 1979 that was the day things started to change for my grandmother. In what looked like a dark world, a leak of light suddenly sprang up and she began to see hope, joy and life. That was the day that I was born and so began the incredible bond that I had with my Grandma Mink.

There are just some people in your life that mean more to you, the ones who you have a special connection to, the ones who can tickle you and make you smile when you are in the foulest of moods; the ones who can encourage you when you think all hope is lost; the ones who you run to when you need comfort and with just a word they can lift you up and make you feel all right with the world.

That's how it was with us, I was her little angel after my grandfather died she recognized me as a gift from God to keep her going.

For a long time after my grandfather's death, she lived with us but one day she got very sick and spent a lot of time at the doctor' s and in the hospital. I remember being afraid, thinking that I would lose her. I was very young at the time and I did not want her to die. We had become so close and I grew to depend on her for so many things. I understood what prayer was then, and I spent a lot of time praying for her and when she got better, I was so grateful and thankful to God for his mercy and healing.

There came a time when my grandmother wanted to be independent, and she left my family home in search of her own place. She did not leave me behind, she took me with her. I suppose my parents realized our closeness and they all agreed that it was a good thing for her as well as me to keep us together. So when my grandmother got her own place she made me a part of it and I was happy to be with her.

These were very happy days for me. We did a lot of things together and she always had time for me and helped to mold me into the man I am today. I know that it is never a good thing to spoil a child, but as the child that was being spoiled, I can truly attest to the fact that at the time of the spoiling, there just does not seem to be anything wrong with it, I enjoyed being the center of her attention and taking advantage of her generosity and favor.

If I wanted anything within reason, my grandmother worked very hard to see to it that I got it. I'm not saying that I was given anything that I wanted, my grandmother was a simple woman and she could not afford a lot of things, but it seemed to me back then that I was happy with humble offerings and my grandma Mink was tickled to make a way for me to have them.

It was there in her home that I came to understand the meaning of comfort food, as my grandmother was a woman who loved to shower me with the foods that I loved.

There were days when I came home from a difficult time at school and she was always there with a snack or a treat to make me feel better. It's amazing how small a problem can become with the tempering of the simplest of things: like a grilled cheese sandwich. I could be frustrated, down on myself and everyone else, with an irritation that could spoil my day and the day of all around me when she would offer me a layer of cheese between two pieces of buttered bread grilled to perfection in a pan, then serve it to me on a plate with a glass of milk. My frustration would melt away with each bite.

There were times when I would feel a sickening sense of rejection, those times when I was teased and made to doubt myself.

I would crawl home and be lost in a consuming pit of agony and self-hatred when she would call me to the table and there waiting for me was a pile of creamy mashed potatoes, whipped with enough love and encouragement to make me forget the woes of my day and know one thing; the hands that made those potatoes loved and believed in me, and at that moment, this was all I needed.

I learned to take a lot of comfort and solace in food back then and at the time I had no regrets. Looking back now I see how it created a complication that aided in my dependence on food for relief and may have paved a way for an unhealthy dependence on food in times of emotional distress.   I know my grandmother meant well and in many ways her dedication to me was shown in the gifts she offered, her words of encouragement, the presents she gave me at special times of the year and often for no special occasion just to show me her affection and undying support of me and of course in the special foods she prepared for me to let me see and feel with certainty that I was without a doubt, most loved.

Chapter 3 - Fighting Obesity

There was no doubt about it, I was growing into being more than a strapping young man with big bones and pure muscle, I was fat, and thanks to my friends at school I was reminded of the fact on a regular basis. To pinpoint how it started, where it came about, I couldn't tell you. All I know is that I was always a big kid, I was always being described as plump, chunky, a 'big boy' and the like.

In my younger days, I didn't take it so hard, but there came a time when I was in Junior High School and working my way into those not so wonderful teen years, I grew to be very leery and quite fearful of the fat label.

Kids aren't always so kind when dealing with someone who's different. It really doesn't matter what the difference is, if you stick out for whatever reason, sometimes the attention it brings to you can be embarrassing and heart wrenching.

I had a lot of things going on with me as a child and as I grew into that period of awkwardness, the time between childhood and teenage, I had a lot of trepidation and fears and I was desperate to fit in. Right about that time, my grandma Mink became extremely ill and had to go into the hospital. My anchor in life was taken away from me at the age of 16 and it tore me up. Once again I was faced with the fears of losing her and I could not bear the thought. Before I was ready to let her go, she was brought to my aunt's house because of her illness as she needed constant care and attention and could not care for herself, much less me.

At this time I moved back into my parents' home and in a short while, my grandmother died leaving me sad and depressed. I was so upset at her passing, I had to look for ways to cope with her loss. I remembered our wonderful times together and how she would do simple and loving things to show me kindness. In time I was making my favorite foods in honor of her and before long, I was blowing up, gaining a lot of weight as a result of my attempts to comfort myself at her loss.

I think it is funny how we use food that way. It is a simple thing with a definite purpose in life but because of our intense need for it, sometimes our desire for it can break off into a passion and many times we fall victim to creating an addiction for it. Like a lot of drugs and enslaving components, food can make us feel good and we are often seduced by its smells, flavors, tastes. When we are looking for a way to feel better, sometimes we go to food and I don't have to tell you that the results are often not favorable. It's a sneaky trap some of us fall into without realizing where we are before we are able to free ourselves from its effects, it is often too late.

I knew I was in trouble with being overweight when I got into high school and after losing my grandmother which caused me to take consolation with food, I learned pretty quickly that I had to gain control over that vice or I would be the laughing stock on campus.

I was already getting teased by a lot of the strong-willed and spirited boys in school and in spite of the fact that I knew they were only kidding and mischievously toying with me, it still hurt and I grew to have a complex. This was the driving force that kept me from losing it with food as a teenager. I had to watch myself, had to control my appetite if I was going to maintain my dignity in those high school years.

It worked and I managed to graduate in 1998 with a smile on my face. But once I got out of high school, the fear of being teased left me and I was faced with an ongoing wave of more than a few of my favorite things. Not afraid of gaining weight anymore and the fear of being made fun of subsided and now I was free to eat as I pleased. I started to get bigger now and my growing size frightened me.

I had a plan. I was going to work on being healthy. I had to because I needed to be a good example to my younger brother, Brandon, who was fifteen years younger than me. In spite of the difference in our age, my brother and I were very close. But like most brothers, we wanted to do things together. We wanted to play ball, take long hikes, go to sports events together and cheer for our favorite teams. But unfortunately, I was in no condition to do any of these things. I had become so large it was difficult to walk a short distance and throwing a ball was possible but even that small effort wore me out. My young brother was full of energy and life and he did not understand why I couldn't do the things that we should have been sharing.

I tried a lot of diets. My mother was very good at dispensing weight loss tips and information. She was very supportive and always encouraged me to do what was necessary to reach my goals. I always started strong, in the beginning of every weight loss attempt. I felt like superman over calories and getting fit. But as the days went on, I lost some of my motivation and always seemed to slip into despair and soon I was staring into a deep hole of failure.

It's never easy being different, and I had difficulty understanding why I was not able to eat my favorite foods without any ill effects. It just didn't seem fair, it made me feel like there was something wrong with me, because no matter how I tried, it seemed as though I just couldn't get over the hump.

While everyone else was meeting for pizza, having stacks of pancakes for breakfast with bacon or sausage and enjoying desserts with their meals, I wanted to join them and not have to wobble away from the table feeling like the long lost white jolly green giant baby.

I struggled with this most of my life and felt as though my situation was not fair; I wanted to be normal, I wanted to be able to eat and drink like everybody else. But I was different, trapped in a body I could not control with a distress in my emotional health that was mounting.

Chapter 4 - Facing My Future

I went into college with confidence and a clear vision of my future. I was studying to be a computer information systems networking specialist and I was feeling pretty good about where I was headed, but I continued to enjoy my favorite foods and often used food to appease my boredom. The weight came on so fast, and like that moth caught in the blaze of disaster in the flame, I did not realize how big I was until I was in a position where I felt like I was too big to find a way of escape.

I was a young man who walked in the shadow of a problem I did not quite understand. I don't know how the situation overcame me, but it did not make it any easier to deal with, and many days when the hours of work and study were complete and I was left alone with my thoughts, I would close the door to my truck, shut out the responsibilities of life, and weep my entire drive home.

More than two-thirds of adults in the United States are considered to be overweight or obese. More than one-third of adults are considered to be obese. More than 1 in 20 have extreme obesity. I was in the 1 in 20, and suffering from extreme obesity. If you asked me how it came about, I would tell you I wasn't sure. I will admit to being heavy my entire life, but to put my finger on where it all began, I can't really say. In my early twenties, I was trapped in a body weighing in at 527 pounds and the ramification of this state was disturbing.

Not necessarily a shy man, I found that the strain life placed upon me was turning me into a recluse. I never left home and when I was forced with going out, I realized that it made me nervous and took me to a new level of tension. Surrounded by a supportive family, I found safety in that net of familiarity and got to the point to where I objected highly to participating in even the easiest social experiences; going to the store, visiting friends, taking in a movie, or dining out. I preferred to just stay home in the confines of the safety my family had become.

In 2000, I got my degree and in just weeks after graduation, I landed a job in Swainsboro, Georgia working as a Tech Support Specialist for an internet company.

I was good at my job, maybe I was too good because when there were problems to be handled and no one else was able to deal with them, they sent them to me. No matter who you are or what you do, stress comes to any job sooner or later. After dealing with many problems and situations that made me want to pull my hair out, I began to have some problems myself. But because of my inability to open up and share with others or ask for help, I quickly spiraled into an emotional soup that left very little room for peace or any semblance of joy.

Right around this time I had some serious bouts with mood swings. I would be happy and hopeful one minute, my eyes on the prize that was my future, living the American dream, finding love, getting married, having a family of my own, and living happily ever after in a house on a hill with a white picket fence. These were the times when I actually believed in myself. I thought I could do anything, but that never stuck around for long. Pretty soon I was waking up with a crummy feeling that I just could not shake. I was down, discouraged, feeling badly about myself and everything around me. I wanted to shake out of it, but no matter how I tried I just seemed to slip further and further into the hole. That's when the depression came--incredible feelings of hopelessness, being so down I could barely see the light or good in any day. I had serious bouts with anxiety as well and I found that it was difficult for me to leave my home without great feelings of distress. I was afraid of everybody and everything, and could almost always depend on a panic attack greeting me if I ever went too far from my home.

There were periods when I suffered from paranoid delusions. They didn't last long, but I was suspicious of everyone and feared they were out to get me. In the fall of 2003, I began to experience symptoms that were disturbing and incredibly alarming. I was hearing voices, they told me odd things, frightening things, distressing things and no matter how much I pushed them out of my head and tried to pretend that they were not there, I fell victim to those terrifying whispers time and time again. It is a daunting and forbidding thing to be alone and know that there is no one in sight but to hear voices warning you, giving you caution and creating a fear that is impossible to shake.

I was losing all interest in day-to-day activities and in spite of my lack of energy, I was having trouble sleeping. My mind was a jumble of ideas and my thoughts seemed to race faster and faster with each day. Most days I experienced a lot of agitation and I was flooded with feelings of worthlessness, shame, and blamed myself for every problem on the planet. My job required me to focus and engage in problem solving, but my thoughts were so jumbled I had trouble thinking much less concentrating.

In November, 2003 I was having a difficult time at work with those auditory hallucinations and no matter how I tried to will them away, they would not stop. The voices started and would not go away. I was experiencing things that were not real or based in reality and nothing anybody offered me in fact or truth made sense to me. I was lost in my delusions. I could not think and soon my behavior was so odd and unusual, I was having trouble communicating with those around me. At one point I actually thought I was a prophet and it was my responsibility to check on the salvation of all of those around me. At this time, my supervisor became alarmed by my behavior and called me into his office to be evaluated.

In a matter of hours I was overtaken by emotional distress and I had a breakdown that summoned the Emergency Squad and took me to the local hospital. Now, you have to understand, our hospital was not the greatest, and I was not happy to be taken there and in my emotional distress, I wandered out into the hallway and let my disapproval be made known. I stood in the middle of that hallway and shouted, "I don't want to be here because this hospital has a bad reputation."

I am not aware of all that occurred that day, but I do know that I had lost it; I was in trouble and so confused and frightened I did not know what to do. So I lied, I told them that I had just had a religious moment, I was moved by the spirit, but now realized that this was inappropriate and apologized for my behavior telling them that I would work very hard to not let it happen again.

Later that night when I was at home with my parents, my behavior was still erratic and my parents thought they needed to get me some help. So they took me back to the local hospital where I was then evaluated by a mental health professional and it was determined that I needed to be transferred to the mental health hospital in Augusta, Georgia.

I was diagnosed with Schizoaffective Disorder, and I was kept in the hospital for one and a half weeks. To say that I was in charge and aware one hundred percent of the time would be a lie. I was out of it and lost in a cloud of confusion and hopelessness. At the time I thought I was a goner. I had little to no optimism for my future.

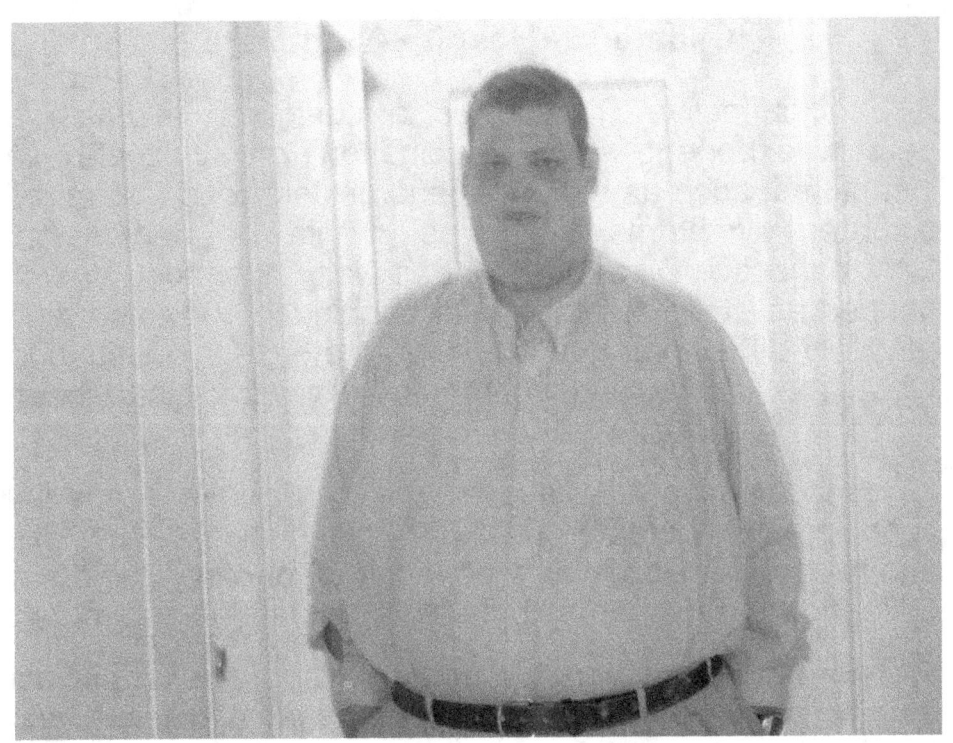

Chapter 5 - Hospital Nightmare

Schizoaffective Disorder is a condition in which a person experiences a combination of schizophrenia symptoms, such as hallucinations or delusions and mood disorder symptoms, such as mania or depression. Schizoaffective Disorder is not as well understood or well defined as other mental health conditions and this made recovery difficult for me, but I was grateful for the support I got from family and church friends once I had been properly diagnosed.

It's one thing to discover that you have a mental condition that creates audible hallucinations, but it's another to be trapped in a hospital full of others who are suffering from the same kinds of hallucinations and more.

The experience was daunting and in spite of the fact that I was suffering from a debilitating mental disorder and heavily medicated, the memories I walked out of that hospital with left an indelible mark in my memory.

People joke about being delusional, someone has a high opinion of themselves, they are told to be delusional. Someone has high expectations about a given situation, they are told to be delusional. But the truth of the matter is being plagued with delusions is no simple or ordinary matter. It is a frightening and incapacitating thing.

Once in the hospital, I was full of fear, seriously confused, and incapable of thinking clearly. It was not clear to me that the medical staff was there to help me. I was certain that everyone was against me and I was doomed to die if I did not get out of that hospital and do it in a hurry.

When I was admitted, they stripped me of everything, including my shoe strings, looking back, I know they were trying to protect, but at the time, I was filled with fear and thinking the worst. Once they had cleared me, they gave

25

me a cup of shampoo and told me to go and wash up. I was convinced that they were trying to kill me and had handed me a cup of poison to finish the job. I was drinking the shampoo to make their job easier when one of the orderlies realized what I was doing and stopped me.

There were physical exams. I saw quite a few doctors who took my vitals and checked my bloodwork. Being poked and prodded in a physical exam is entirely different than being studied and scrutinized with a mental magnifying glass. I was asked questions that I couldn't answer, I reacted badly and I soon discovered that it was better for me to remain quiet than to say anything at all.

For the first two or three days as they evaluated me, I was with no medication because they wanted to see how I behaved without meds. I would go to the med cart when it rolled in hoping they had something for me as I was feeling a bit left out on the medication train. Once I was properly diagnosed, however, they prescribed medications and I was soon on a daily regime of medications.

The medication I was given was not always pleasant and there were days when I felt nervous and sick and others when I had trouble feeling anything at all. The nurses and orderlies were just doing their jobs, I tried to understand this, but I often saw them as my enemies and was convinced that they were more like prison guards than medical professionals.

Every time I went into a room the door was locked behind me. If I sat down to have a meal, the door was locked. If I was led into a room for recreation, they locked me in. If I had an appointment with a doctor I was locked into the room with him. When I had a visitor, it was difficult to see it as a good experience because I felt like a prisoner who had to be locked away in every situation. I never got used to the hospital lockdowns and with each day I grew more and more weary of it and would often dream of escaping and making my way back to my home where I was surrounded by my family and a safety net of friends.

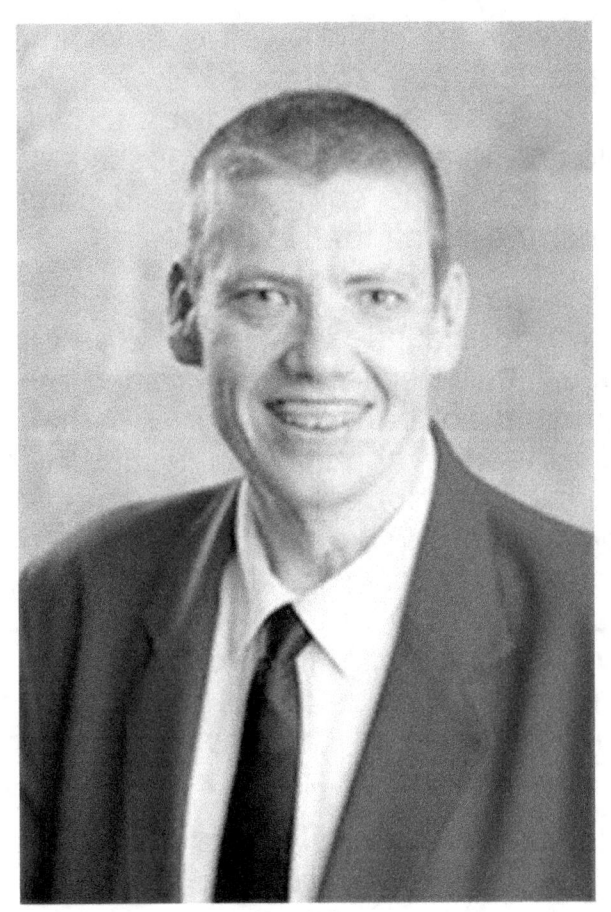

There were times when I was overwhelmed with fear and frightened beyond compare by what was going on around me. I was paranoid and given to delusions and I was not alone, there were so many locked away with me who were suffering the same fate, and some who I felt were so much worse off than I was.

One day I was approached by a man who appeared to be a kind and gentle fellow. We entered into a conversation, and in spite of our strained environment, I felt like he might not be a bad sort. But that was before he started to tell me about his collection of needles he had mounting in his room. He had thousands of them, all over the place and he was desperate to keep it a secret. He warned me to not disclose this information to anyone, not the other patients, not the nurses or the orderlies. After my conversation with him, I couldn't wait to get back to my room because I was certain that I was safer alone than around this sort of thing which I was convinced would certainly prove to be my doom.

The orderlies were strong and reliable men who did not hesitate to secure a room and keep everyone settled and in calm behavior. I discovered all too quickly that I should not mess with them and if they told me to do something it was easier to just comply; I could not question them, refuse or even hesitate as they were quick to enforce their commands. If any of the patients challenged their orders, they were swiftly taught a lesson in the importance of obeying and if someone got out of line, misbehaved or simply tried to walk out, the orderlies were on it.

I witnessed a man who was foolish enough to challenge their authority once. He was without a doubt suffering from instability and not in charge of himself and rebelled against what he was told to do. He was going into the laundry room and searching people's laundry looking for money. His intention was not good and he meant to steal what he had found. The orderlies went after him and what ensued was not a pretty sight; he was subdued and not in a very pleasant fashion. A few orderlies rushed into the situation with brute force and before the patient was rendered restrained and submissive, they had tossed him around the room and at one point thrown him over a sofa.

I was terrified after seeing such things and was praying for God to deliver me and let me go home. I did not feel like I belonged there, I wanted to get back to my family, my house in Midville where I could feel safe and comfortable again. One day seemed like a year in that place and I thought if I stayed there another day I would never get better, only worse.

One day my parents came to visit me and I was so happy to see them. I don't remember everything that occurred that day during that visit but I am sure I let them know how unhappy I was and how desperate I was to get out of there. They were as wonderful as they always were, telling me I was going to be okay, I'd get out of there soon but first I had to get the medical attention I needed and I had to be brave and understand that it was for the best.

At the moment I was not brave, I was frightened and worried that I would never get out of there. I felt like I had been in there long enough, I felt like I was only getting worse staying in there and having to be locked away. I didn't like the orderlies and the way they treated people, I feared them and wondered when they would pick on me and possibly man-handle me and try to throw me over a sofa.

When my parents were saying their goodbyes, I decided that it was good a time as any to make my move. When they walked past the locked door that led to freedom, I did my best to go with them. I didn't try to sneak, I didn't push my way past security, I just followed them and hoped no one would notice. But they noticed, not just one but a few orderlies came racing to the scene to pull me back into the locked arena they called a hospital and I did not go quietly. I pushed against them, trying to get back to my parents and they pulled me all the harder. I tried to convince them that it was alright for me to leave, I thought they should listen to me, hear me out and then hopefully let me go, but it was a no-go. Once they'd gotten me pinned down, someone came flying to the scene with a hypodermic needle full of a sedative and in minutes I blacked out.

When I awoke, it was some time later and I was in a room by myself feeling groggy and somewhat disconnected. It took only a minute for me to remember what had happened and at the thought of it all, I felt such a rush of hopelessness. The tears began to come as I laid there feeling like a lost cause and I wondered if I would ever get out of that place.

Chapter 6 - Moving On

Finally, the day I'd been hoping for, praying would happen did and I was released from the hospital. That was a happy day for me but somewhat bittersweet. I was happy to be released, happy to be going home to be with my family and in a familiar, friendly atmosphere where I felt safe, but I was leaving the hospital with a label, I was suffering with Schizoaffective Disorder, and I was told I would have to take medication to control it the rest of my life.

I was still having symptoms, but when someone asked me how I was doing I told them I was fine, I was completely recovered. I pretended to be normal, safe, free of all indicators of the disorder and I was anxious to reassume my place in society once again.

But the truth of the matter was that I was still experiencing signs of the disorder, I was still hearing voices and I was still very afraid for myself and my situation. Once I got home, I did not want to leave. I felt safe there, I did not have to worry about orderlies or nurses or doctors pulling me into a room and giving me the third degree. I got to the point to where I was afraid to leave home, it was much worse than before now and the thought of having to go somewhere terrified me.

I had a follow up appointment with my doctor but I did not want to go, so I made excuses and found a reason not to. This really hurt me more than it helped me because missing the appointment meant not getting the refills for my medication that I needed and when I called the doctor's office to try to get a refill sent to my pharmacy, my prescribing doctor was not available so instead of trying to find what medication I was needing, they just prescribed me a new one. It was not doing a very good job, and soon I found myself with no energy, sleepy all of the time and quite lethargic. I did not complain, however, I was afraid to, I thought that if I told somebody how badly I was feeling they might load me up in an ambulance and take me back to the hospital. I did not want to go back, so I pretended everything was fine.

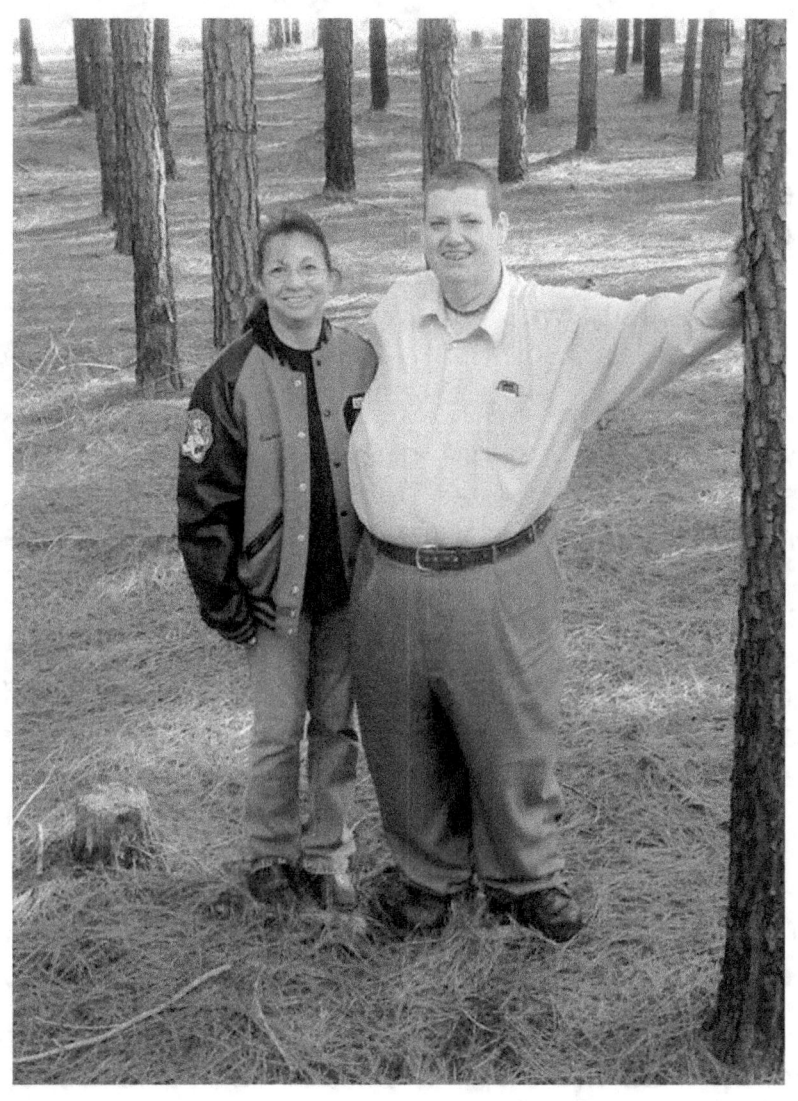

One day I accompanied my mother to town to do some errands and to see her doctor and when he saw me he told her that he was not sure that the medications I was on were doing such a good job. In his estimation, I looked like a zombie, and told her to have me reevaluated as soon as possible. I did not like the sound of this and found myself spiraling into a panic, I argued, told her I was fine, nothing was wrong, I was just tired from all I'd been through, but she didn't listen, she trusted her doctor and insisted that I see a psychiatrist.

When I was evaluated by a new psychiatrist, I pretended everything was good, I was not honest at all when he asked me questions and lied about my situation. He was a smart doctor, and would not let up until he was satisfied as to what was really going on with me. I finally owned up to my fibbing and told him that I was afraid of being sent back to the hospital. He told me he was there to help me, and did not want me to go back to the hospital either. He assured me that if he was going to help me and give me the proper medication to control the illness and keep me out of the hospital, I had to be honest with him. From that point on, I told the truth and he was able to find a medication that took care of my symptoms and helped me to walk through my life without complications.

Like all who have been given the label of a debilitating disorder, I had regrets and a lot of self-doubt. I wanted the freedom to stand on my own, but the truth was that I was not only suffering mentally, I had quite a few physical problems going on as well. At this point I was over five hundred pounds and I could not do a lot of the things I wanted to do or needed to do. I was somewhat immobile and simple things like walking to the front door, riding in an automobile, pushing a grocery cart through the store-- all easy and necessary activity in a day to day life, but I found it difficult and nearly impossible to do.

I soon discovered that I was incapable of taking care of myself and began to explore my options. I had several serious physical problems that made life somewhat difficult for me. Besides the mental disability, the toll of health problems and risks were mounting and I knew I needed help with personal care and for the wounds I was suffering from. I had ulcers all around my lower legs and it was difficult for me to care for them the way I needed to.

After a visit to my family physician's office in July of 2009, my doctor helped me come to a conclusion. I knew that I could not care for myself and I did not want to put the burden of my care on anyone in my family. It was not an easy decision to make, but at the age of 26, I checked myself into a nursing home to assure that I had the care that I needed with a goal of losing 100 pounds before being discharged.

I had 2 therapists, a physical therapist and an occupational therapist. I remember the physical therapist fondly, because he was what I call a 'godsend'.

He gave me the motivation I needed to forget about the obstacles before me and to just start moving towards my goal.

One of the most difficult things for me to face during the two years I was in the nursing home was the fact that I was just 26 years old in a home full of older people and many with mental and physical disabilities. I tried to keep myself occupied during this time, and stayed focused on my goal.

The obstacles in my way were many times overwhelming and I found it difficult to center my attention and energies on fixing myself. I knew that the burden of my recovery was lying on me and I was determined to make a strong effort to get the work done that I knew needed to be accomplished. This was not always easy and there were times when I felt lost, alone and not at all capable of fulfilling the work necessary to fix my problems and pull me through my dilemma. There were times when I messed up; I faltered and fell and I wondered if I would ever be strong enough to get up and start again. These were very trying times for me, it's not like I had a wealth of confidence and a steady stream of self-esteem, I doubted myself and was often overcome by fears and trepidation.

I had a lot of help from the staff at the nursing home and of course my family and close friends were always encouraging me and motivating me to move on. I found comfort in their belief in me and I knew that the power of God was at work in me and would not fail me. I marched on in my battle to save myself.

After two years, I felt like I had come close to fulfilling my promise to myself and had managed to complete half of my objective, I lost 50 pounds. I was disappointed to not be able to lose the entire 100 pounds but as time went on I discovered that I was making some positive changes and I thought I was ready to move on to a new phase in my recovery.

Once out of the nursing home, I thought I would continue with my weight loss regime, but the pressure of life and the constant availability of my favorite foods were too much for me to handle. In the nursing home I had a lot of structure, the help of a dietitian, physical therapists who pushed me to move and work out. At home, I was free to sit and watch television, I was not moving as much as I should have been and pretty soon I was falling into old habits. In a short time, I'd gained twenty of the fifty pounds back. Determined to get back on track, I began to explore my options and found myself at a cardiologists office with the hope that this doctor would give me the help I needed by recommending that I have weight loss surgery.

I remember the visit well. Living in a small town in South Georgia, there was no local cardiologists, however one came down to satisfy the needs of the rural community and I had an appointment. Sitting in that office was enough of a nerve racking experience, but once the doctor came in and took a look at me, things got even worse.

When the doctor was finished with the examination, he stood back and declared, "Oh, boy, you're really fat, aren't you?"

It was a forthright and all-too-blunt statement, and in spite of knowing that it was in all honesty a truth, it did not make the pain of facing that unpretentious and direct fact any easier. I felt awful; my feelings were hurt, and I was humiliated.

Thankfully, the cardiologist saw the need for weight loss surgery and his recommendation made it possible for me to be approved but I would have to lose 40 pounds before the surgery could take place. So now I had to put myself in gear and make the 40 pound loss a reality and at this point I was ready to do whatever I had to do to make it happen. I knew that I could count on my mother. She would help me with the food. She pointed me to salads, but for some reason I had an aversion to salads, so we had to go another route. I ate lots of fresh vegetables but the key to my success was portion control. I also knew I could depend on my family to help me, they would encourage me, motivate me, and help me get the strength that I needed to do what I had to do.

This was pretty much a life and death situation, and I had already realized that I was tired of living the way I had been. One problem melted into the other and as I tried to find a way to fix myself, I knew that I could lean on the healthy support system that was made up by family and close friends.

I did in fact meet my 40 pound goal and went over it by 60 pounds, having lost 100 pounds, I felt successful and ready for my life. Finally after years of self-doubt and lack of confidence that my extreme obesity had caused me most of my life, I was feeling positive and well on my way to reclaiming my life.

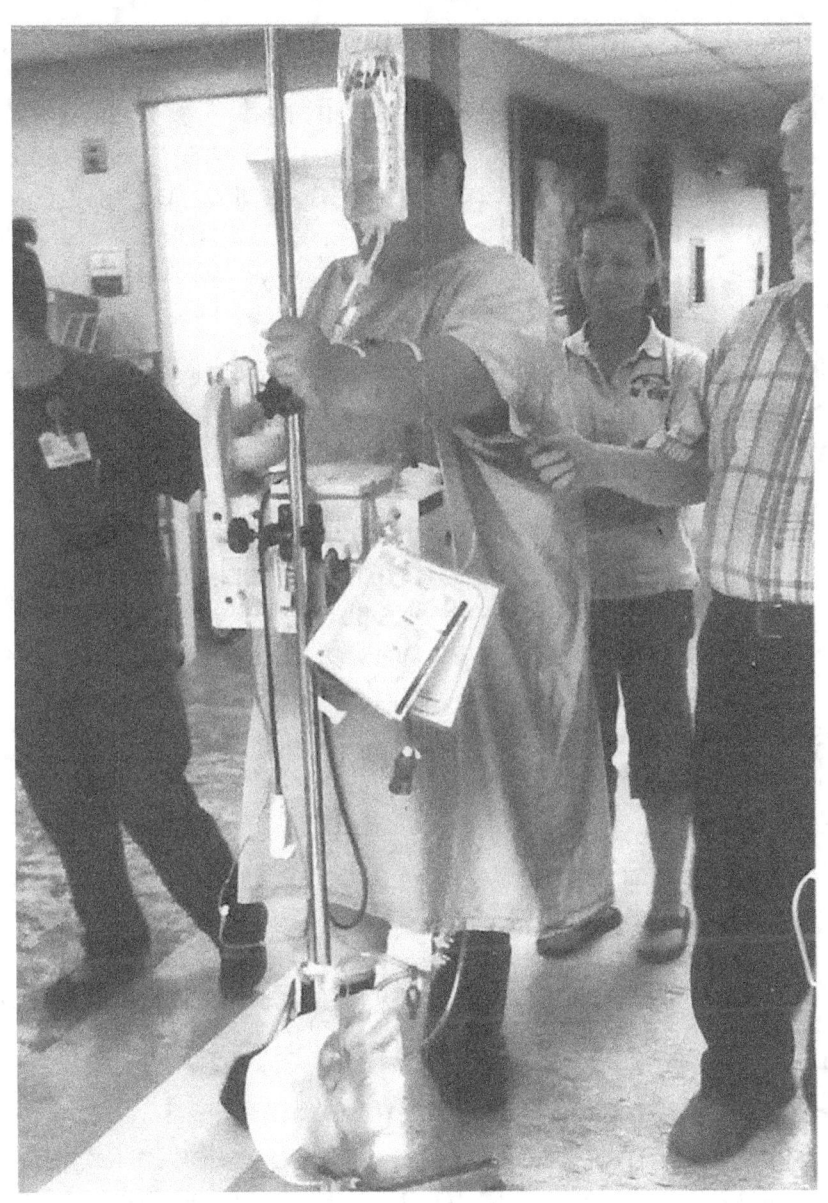

Chapter 7 - Independence Day

Maybe I did not lead a sheltered life, but being a country boy living in a small town in southern Georgia, my adventures were limited and in spite of my health problems, mentally and physically, I had never really been sick enough to have to have surgery, so the thought of being cut on and opened up frightened me.

I knew weight loss surgery was necessary, I knew it was going to change my life. I knew without it I would keep falling and failing and sooner or later I would have to live in a nursing home and be cared for because I would not be able to survive on my own. I had a lot of things going on in my head as I moved towards weight loss surgery, I questioned the procedure, I worried about being put to sleep and of course I was afraid that I would die on the operating table. I don't think this is so unusual, I think most people having any kind of surgery go through this and the trepidation can be daunting and a bit overwhelming.

Preparing for surgery was a busy time. I had a lot of doctor visits and medical procedures. I was told that I would have to jump through a lot of hoops to be approved for surgery, but once I had my surgery date I was full of mixed emotions. Finally, I was going to have the surgery that I knew would change my life for the better. I was going to lose weight, get healthy and start enjoying my life. On the other hand, I was going to be checked into the hospital, I was going to be prepped for surgery and I was going to have anesthesia. I tried to not think about the actual surgery, it had been explained to me and I knew what was going to happen, but in spite of the words of encouragement I was hearing from my friends and family, in spite of the fact that I knew my doctor was a skilled surgeon and he had done this procedure many times, I was still frightened.

I remember the day I checked into the hospital, trembling and full of anxiety, I had one very big rock to stand on; I knew God was with me, and if He was on my side, it did not matter what I came against. I kept remembering scriptures and repeating them to myself, I knew that I could do this, because Christ enabled me to do all things. My parents were praying, my friends were praying and thankfully, I had a surgeon who was a Christian who would not let me go under anesthesia until he prayed with me, so I was feeling pretty blessed as they rolled me into the Operating Room.

Before I went under, my doctor told me to remember something. He said when you are awake, you need to realize that the best and healthiest way to recover is to start walking as soon as you can after surgery. He assured me that this was best, and when I came to consciousness in the recovery room I remembered his words. I came through the surgery with flying colors and I was at peace with the knowledge of knowing that because I had praying friends and family, I was blessed with success.

Two hours later, I was up and walking. Not everybody is so quick to move into walking after surgery but I was determined to put a move on my recovery and obey doctor's orders, so I went to work. I must tell you, it was not an easy thing. I was in a lot of pain and very groggy from the anesthesia and pain meds but I was unwavering to follow doctors' orders and succeed so I pushed myself to compliance.

I have photos of me taking my first steps after surgery and when I look at those pictures I remember the steady determination I felt and I have to smile. I had felt defeated, wounded and damaged most of my life and here I had been given a chance to take care of the problem. I was not going to blow it.

With every step I was fortified with courage and power, I was doing it, working towards my future and I knew without a doubt that I would succeed and be a better man.

When I got home from the hospital, it was July 4, 2012. This was a most distinctive day for me because I knew it was a pivotal time. I told my family and friends that this was the day I was declaring my independence from this unhealthy lifestyle that I had been living. I made a quality decision that day, to move on and become the man I was meant to be and I was convinced that I could move on and do exactly that. It was hard not to remember just three years earlier when I was admitted to the Heritage Healthcare Nursing Home in Swainsboro in 2009. What a difference three years had made.

I followed my doctor's orders and walked every day as much as I possibly could. I was also diligent with drinking water and four ounce shots of protein shakes which was necessary for my success. It being necessary did not make it easy, and I had lots of problems pushing those fluids down, but I pushed through and with the grace of God I was very successful.

Before weight loss surgery, I had type 2 diabetes and I was on medication for it, I took Glucophage pills daily. I had sleep apnea and had to sleep with a mask and a Bipap machine. After weight loss surgery, I was amazed to discover that I no longer needed to use the Bipap machine with oxygen. I could sleep alone in my bed without the tubes, the noise and that spooky mask. I was also given the clear on the diabetes. No more Glucophage pills for me, I was free of that medication and not having any more Type 2 Diabetes symptoms. It is an amazing thing to discover how much of a difference just the surgery would make, but telling you this gives me reason to smile big, because the changes and effects brought on by weight loss surgery go much further and bring so many wonderful life-altering events and as the months went on in 2012 and 2013, I discovered that my life was full of delightful surprises.

I had a friend who had had weight loss surgery prior to me, his name was Phillip and he was a big support to me during this time of change.

He had found a sale on Treadmills and when he took home his purchase, he did not just carry one machine from the store, he had two; one for him and one as a gift to me. He met my uncle in Augusta, while I was recovering from surgery and helped load that treadmill into my uncle's vehicle and sent it to me with his well wishes. This is just one of the events that took place in my life at this time that makes me believe more and more in the miracles of God and I feel extremely blessed because of them.

It only took me a few week to get to feeling well enough to want to start working on a serious fitness program. I joined the CPR gym and found a trainer, Mr. Robert Allen. Mr. Robert has taken me on an incredible journey from a fat, fluffy unhappy man of 527 pounds through hills and valleys, mud holes and bumps. Times when I wondered if I was strong enough, days when I thought I would never catch my breath again. The beginning was tough, but I was told that if I wanted to gain health and grow stronger, it would not be easy, but the results would be so worth it.

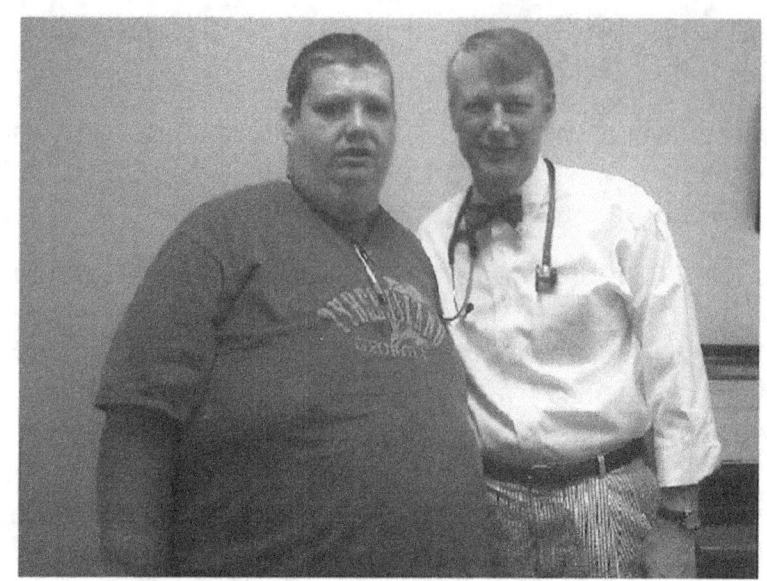

Me and Dr. Edward Boland Medical Weight Loss Doctor

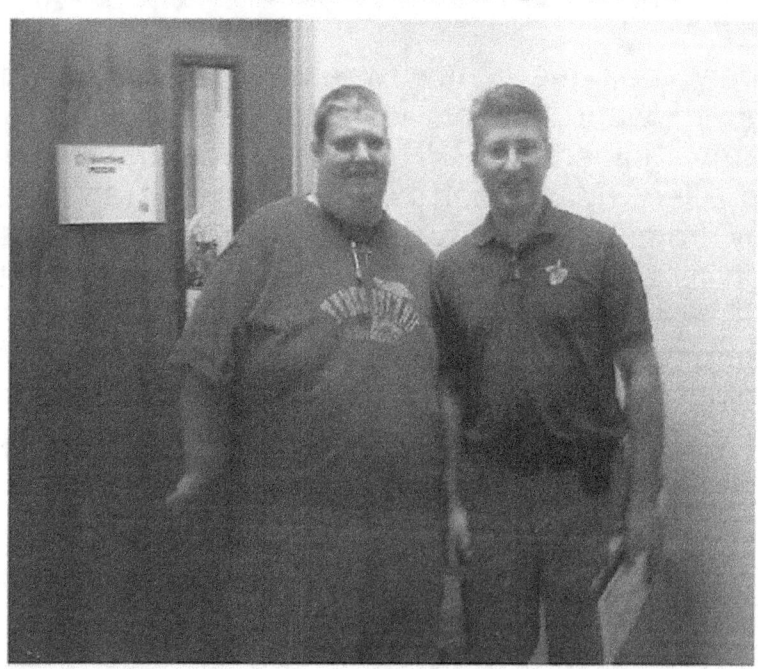

Me and Dr. Darren Glass Bariatric Surgeon

I pressed forward, determined to make a difference and as I did the pounds began to fall off and I felt something in me that I had never really experienced before, muscles and strength! I worked out daily on the treadmill, lifting weights, walking--and in time I saw an incredible difference. I will tell you that working out at 500 pounds is no easy task, but as you move past the awkwardness, the inability to move, the impossibility of agility and flexibility--evolution comes and you begin to see remarkable things. I remember the first time I was able to work out without losing my breath, the first time I was able to lift a lot of weight without winching and on the day that I was able to squat without running into flab, I was one happy man.

My trainer tailored an exercise program specifically to meet my needs, he knew where I was and where I wanted to be and was able to lead me on a voyage of improvement and immense discovery. As I grew stronger and more agile, he adjusted the program continuing to challenge my endurance and strength until I was feeling like a seasoned athlete.

Another thing that really helped me in my progress with weight loss was joining a support group to help me with my eating and food. I joined a Weight Watchers Group in Swainsboro. I needed to be accountable with my weight, and they helped me to do that. I went to weekly classes under the direction and guidance of Mrs. Theresa Proctor and I was very happy with my achievement there.

There is something to be said about being accountable. A lot of people think they can do it on their own, they don't need anybody's help and for the most part they push forward and do alright. But I am a firm believer that people need to check themselves to be able to ask for help when needed. I had that problem in my early days and was incapable of asking for help and it got me into a lot of trouble, but when I had surgery things changed and I realized I was not an island and I needed to reach out for a helping hand now and again.

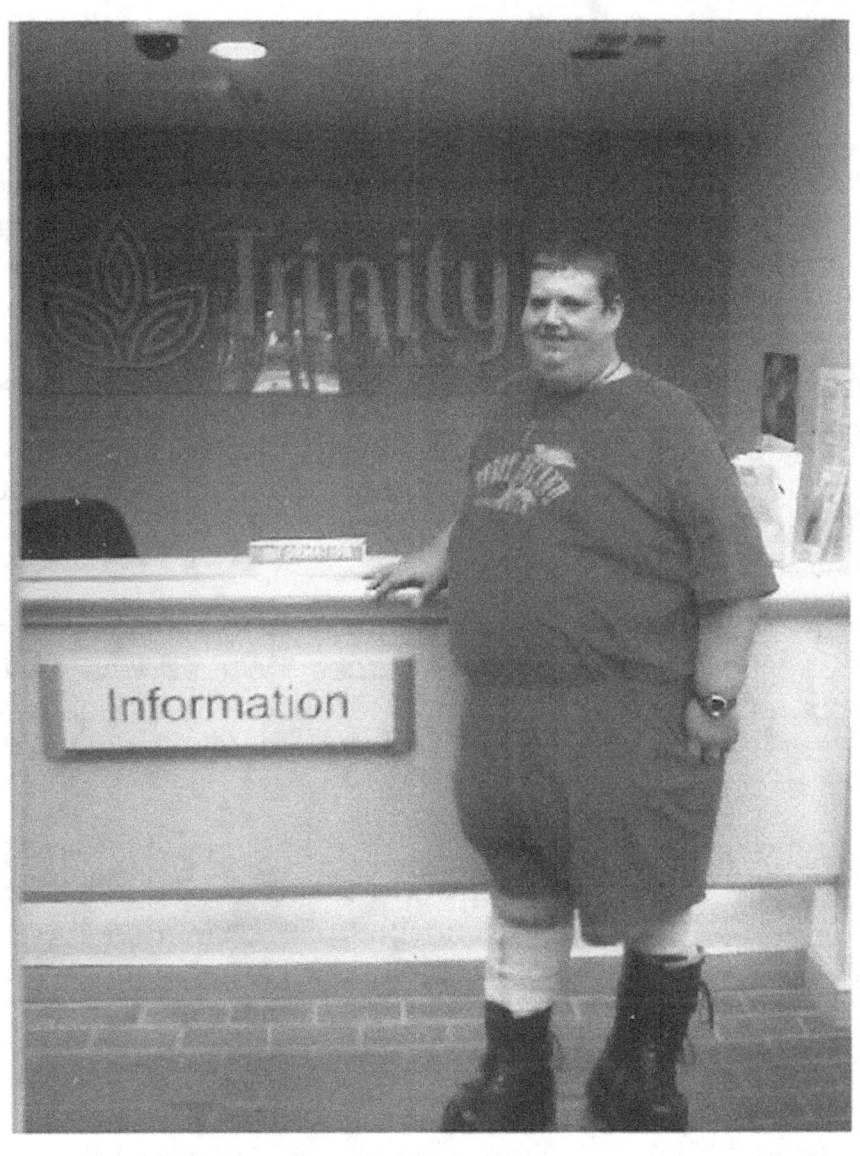

Me at Trinity Hospital Day of Surgery July 3, 2012

When you work with a weekly support group the way I did, you not only get an ongoing record of your weight and progress, but you get a weekly boost. The classes at Weight Watchers really helped me to put things into prospective. I learned how to cope with every day issues and was assured that I was not the only one feeling stress or pressure. I was educated on nutrition and learned so much about what was healthy and what was not. I also got great advice on things like portion control, unhealthy food triggers and how to prevent binges and mindless eating.

Mrs. Proctor proved to be an incredible leader and I soon discovered that she was a great source of motivation and inspiration.

She was always there, making herself available to me for questions, advice and resources. When I was feeling discouraged she would send me encouraging postcards in the mail and when I received them, I would always find such encouragement.

I am so very grateful for the people God put into my life during my time of healing and my journey to health and wellness. It is a comforting thing to know that there is always a silver lining on every dark cloud that comes into our lives and no matter what, we can always find a way to a happy life.

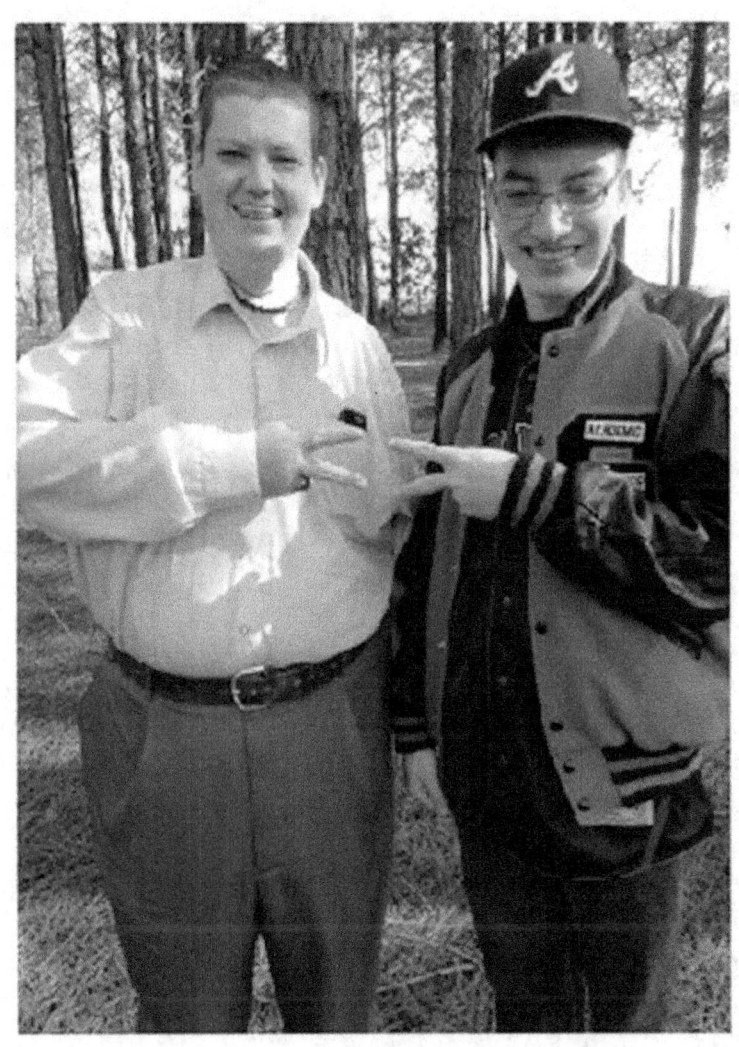

Me and my Brother Brandon

Chapter 8 - Changes

They say change is good, but when you are obese living under layers of fat, change is something you dream about, but once you are faced with the possibility, you tend to doubt yourself. Will this diet work? Will I be able to stay on this weight loss plan? Will I be able to stay away from the sweets, the pizza, the ice cream, the greasy hamburgers? Self-doubt plagues every dieter I think, I mentioned before how motivated I was in the beginning of every weight loss plan and how at first I felt like I was going to make it, succeed and lose many sizes in a year, but as time went on I was hit by doubt and fear and many times I think it was that doubt and fear that paralyzed me and kept me from being a success.

I think what happens to the fat person many times is we know the solutions, we know what we have to do to get out of the hole we are in but in many ways we are afraid of the changes that are necessary to take us from misery to success. It may sound strangely peculiar, but the truth is we get comfortable where we are, in many ways we are miserable, but in just as many ways we feel safe and don't want to move for fear of messing up and making our condition worst. This is what I mean by the fear that paralyzes us, we know we have to move, but we are afraid to fail, so we stay where we are in the safety of the same old same old.

Many times I think it takes something drastic for us to make the move towards change, it is the only way we are rocked into the reality of our situation and as we are faced with the dilemma of facts, we find the motivation to move, and many times that motivation is fear. That's when we push ourselves to fix ourselves and it is never easy, especially when you are immobile, sedentary; like a fixture on the sofa.

There were times when I saw the walk to the bathroom as a long hike, twenty or thirty steps and it was like an Olympic event for me. There were times when I put off going to the kitchen to get a drink of water, when the phone rang I was hating to get up to go answer it and to go and get the mail from the mail box was something I would put off whenever I could, it was so hard and physically exerting.

I was a couch vegetable. My main activities involved me on my bottom, watching television, playing video games. I would even have to sit in a chair when I played sports with my young brother. Was I happy in that state? No, of course not, I was miserable and sometimes I would get desperate and full of anxiety over my condition and I would pray and beg God for mercy. It's a miserable thing to sit still while life is whirling past you, to know that you are incapable of doing the simplest things.

Even when I would go out, I was sitting; sitting in my handicap scooter when I went to the store, sitting in my handicap scooter when I went to the mall, or the park.

I could not shop unless I used one of those electric carts and if I had to get things and there was none available, I would have to sit on a bench and wait for one to come back and if they were not available, I had to go home without doing the shopping I had to do.

Travel was impossible. The only way I could get around was in my large full size Chevrolet Sierra, the biggest truck they make was the only way I could get about. If I wanted to travel a long distance, I had to drive or just forget about it because I could not fit in a bus seat or a train seat and flying on an airplane was out of the question.

Who doesn't like going to fairs and festivals? Of course I did and my family would make it a fun experience, but I could not walk around I had to depend on the scooter to get me around and it was impossible to get on any of the rides. I just had to enjoy the day's events from my chair and pretend it didn't bother me. But it did, it bothered me a lot.

In many ways I felt like a man trapped in a hole. I wanted to climb out and enjoy life, but no matter how much I tried, I just could not get out of that hole. I would hear friends and family talking about going to Southern Georgia sporting events, baseball, football, basketball. I would listen intently to the stories about the excitement, wishing with all of my might that I could do it, get in the car and drive down to the stadium or the sports arena and sit in the stands wearing my team's colors and cheering for my squad. It was only a dream, however, and it depressed me sometimes. I wanted so badly to be able to walk, run and fit into those little seats and enjoy sporting events, but I was never able to.

When I had weight loss surgery I knew that it was going to create a need for drastic changes in my life and as ready as I was for the changes, I doubted that I could carry it out. I had a lot of fear and trepidation and I wondered if it was going to work. I'd heard of others who had had the surgery and lost 100 pounds only to gain it back. Was that going to happen to me? Until my preparation for weight loss surgery, I had never really been successful at losing weight and I found myself fearing failure and doubting myself a lot.

Another thing that a lot of people don't realize is not just the fat person's dependence on food, but his love for it. I had a serious love affair with Little Debbie Cakes and peanut butter cups. There were days, bad days when I would feel frustrated, hurt and annoyed and the only thing that had the power to get me out of that unpleasant mood was my sweet snacks. Like a favorite person who comes in to make you feel better, the one who has that special power over you to make you forget your troubles and find

53

a smile, Little Debbie Cakes and Peanut Butter Cups did that for me and I was afraid that I would not be able to make it without them.

My social life was not very social, I was in no physical condition to enjoy going to the movies with my friends or out to a concert. One of my most embarrassing moments happened in the theater, I went with some friends to see a movie. Finding a seat was easy, fitting in it was not. I made it through the movie but when it was time to get up and go, I broke the seat. I did not do it quietly, you know so no one knew what had happened. It was noisy and obvious and I was so embarrassed by what had happened, I could not wait to get out of there. That was when I made up my mind that I could not go to the movies. I never wanted to suffer that embarrassment again.

As far as relationships went, I always liked girls and wanted to have a relationship. When I was in high school I had a girlfriend and I thought we had a good relationship. We spent a lot of time together and enjoyed our time together until one day I was at her house and heard her mother talking about me. I knew she did not like me and was never really certain why until this particular day when she was talking to her daughter about me.

She was not happy with her daughter, was telling her how she was settling for something she did not deserve and if she would just do something to help herself, change herself, she could lose some weight and find a boyfriend who was worth something and better suited for her. What she was saying was that I was a big boy, too fat and not good enough for her daughter. It was a terribly painful thing to go through and I tried to move past it, but it still stabs at my feelings today.

One of my favorite things to do was go to church. I loved worshiping God and spending time with the Christians at my church. It was not always easy for me to join in on church activities, but they always tried to include me and I did enjoy our fellowship together. There came a time when I felt like God was calling me to be a preacher, I was excited about this, but soon discovered that my condition prevented me from following through with any serious ministry. I could not stand behind the pulpit for more than a minute at a time and no sermon is instantaneous. I felt like I was supposed to be delivering hour sermons on the wonders of God and I could barely spell out a minute of testimony. This was frustrating and I wanted very much to do what I needed to do to change this.

I can't really remember having any confidence about any given thing in my life back then. I remember seeing confidence in other people and wishing for it, wanting it, thinking that I could be confident about something, but what? I'd dig into myself to try to find the confidence and self-assurance to stand and say I believed in myself. I knew I could do it, but the truth was, I had none. I had friends with poise and grace and I wanted it, too. I was told by a lot of people that I might not have confidence in myself, but I could be confident in the fact that God had created me to do wonderful things. I tried to believe that, I tried to hang on to scripture and have the faith to know that I was strong and secure in my Lord, but even then I had difficulty.

I tried to hold on to the truth of God's Word every day and I knew that He was at work in me willing and doing His good pleasure. I knew that things were happening quickly after weight loss surgery and I was seeing some real results. I remember feeling like I was in the middle of a miracle and it was an extraordinary thing and I could see and realize things that I had once only dreamed of.

I felt the changes taking place and I was excited about the possibilities. I thought about the little sparrow that flies about the earth searching for sustenance. They don't have to worry, they don't have to make things happen, they just have to trust God.

I knew without a doubt that this is what I had to do. I had to forget the results, forget the food I was missing, the exercise I was going to have to do and just trust God.

Making changes is never an easy thing, but once you make up your mind that change is a good thing and it is well worth your effort to climb out of that hole, that rut that you dug for yourself for so many years and found comfort in it.

Once you find the strength to move on and follow through on your commitments, you will find the courage to move into the lane of change and quickly excel to the heights in life that you once could only dream of.

I went through many changes as I ventured through my weight loss journey but there were times when I felt as though I was going to fail, not make it, fall on my face. It is never a pleasant thing to fail but I have found that if we don't fail, if we don't lose our grip on reality and understand that it is a process; a day to day thing and there are no guarantees, we will never make any progress. Once we learn this important lesson, I think we can relax and stop pushing ourselves to be perfect and when the weak moments come we can cut ourselves a little slack and realize that if we don't fall, we can't get up. If we don't fail, we will never experience to joy of victory.

There is a lot to learn from being so overweight that it changes your life, the simple things in life become difficult and in many circumstances we are robbed of the ability to be independent and simple dignity is stripped from us. But as we plow forward in the avenues of change, we make a way to change the things that were once thought impossible into those little rocks of hope that ring true in the realm of impossibility.

The now kind of faith is the substance of things hoped for, the evidence of things not seen quite yet. As I lingered in my morbidly obese state, I had a lot of hope; hope for walking and being active, hope for being able to travel in more than just my big truck. I hoped to be able to play sports with my brother and be a spectator at sporting events. I hoped for a time when I could stand behind the pulpit not just at my church, but in many churches as the Lord sent me forth, to preach about His goodness and grace. I hoped for health and happiness and I hoped for peace and satisfaction in my life. As I walked through the changes that weight loss surgery helped to bring in my life, I began to experience the now and realized that my faith was working and I was beginning to see the evidence of things I had only once dreamed of.

Chapter 9 - A New Chance at Life

If you think about it, 310 pounds is an obese man, according to the insurance charts and the information you might get at your doctor's office, if you signed in at 310 pounds, you'd be considered obese and told to lose some weight. That is how much weight I lost in a span of three years, and when I think about it today, it still blows my mind.

Once I had weight loss surgery things began to happen and I experienced rapid weight loss in the first year. When you read about weight loss surgery and you get an idea of what to expect, it can be exciting, the possibilities, the prospects seem all too amazing and I was eager to see these things in my life, but when it all started to happen, I was more than excited, I was animated with the adventure of it all.

As the months went on that first year, I couldn't wait to get on the scale to see the difference in my body. I lost over a hundred pounds that first year and it was an amazing feeling. I ate very little, small portions and worked hard at exercising and staying active. The first time I got on an elliptical machine I felt like I was going to pass out from the exertion, I could not make sixty seconds it was so difficult for me, but today I own my own elliptical machine and I am on that thing for thirty minutes now.

After the first year, my weight loss began to slow down and I started to experience some discouragement, but that was quickly remedied with the help of my trainer who told me I just had to adjust my workout schedule. I was very eager to comply and as I did, I discovered that the weight began to move off once again.

One of the most disheartening things in any weight loss journey is the pit stops, the times when the weight loss eases up and altogether stops. It's easy to lose hope in those times, we get frustrated and have feelings of failure. I can't really explain what happens in a weight loss stall, but I can tell you this, it is not the time to ease up and ease up on your work to see results, in fact, during those plateaus, it's most important for us to focus and work harder to get through it and to success once again.

I have seen a lot of people get annoyed with the stalls and fizzle out, motivation disappears and the need to be comforted enters. People get frustrated, irritated, aggravated and think the only solution sometimes is to fall back into old habits, and that is the worst thing to do because all it does is creates the original problem that sent you on a weight loss quest in the first place.

The best thing to do when weight loss slows down is to examine your situation; are you eating more? Are you skipping your workouts? If the answer is yes to either of these questions you need to slap yourself out of it and get back on track. Fix your food intake, get back to eating healthy meals, keep your portion control in check and don't add those condiments and sweets that you know are detrimental to your success.

If you are slacking in your exercise program, take the time to figure out where the problem is and move towards changing it. Maybe you think you don't have time to work out, but you have time to watch television and play video games, so the spare time element is in the works and you need to realize that inserting a thirty minute window into your leisure time is not only going to help your weight loss success, it's going to improve your sense of self-esteem. Turn the television on, but instead of flopping down on the sofa, get on that exercise bike, the treadmill or the elliptical machine and crank out a workout. When you get on the scale that month, you'll be glad you did.

In my roughest times during my weight loss journey, I found myself looking for my friends, Debbie and Reese, to pull me out of my funk and make me feel better about where I was. I told you I loved those two guys and having to give them up was tough, especially when I was feeling sad, discouraged, defeated. I knew they had the power to rev me up and make me want to dance. The problem with Debbie and Reese is that once you partake of them, you have to dance for about 2 hours non-stop to work off the calories they put into you. I discovered all too quickly after weight loss surgery that I did not want to go back to that little circle of friends, they were not safe and I knew that would be a bad influence on me. It was not easy, but I said goodbye to Debbie and Reese, I made up my mind that it would not be worth it for me to hang out with them the way I had been accustomed to doing in my past. I did not want to get back to the way I was at 500 plus pounds so I learned to adapt; instead of Reese and Debbie, I made friends with a fellow by the name of Adkins, this guy makes great low carb, high protein bars that taste pretty good and help eliminate my sugar cravings. He and I are great friends now, we get along just fine.

Rough spots are going to come in weight loss and no matter how you try to make them go away and disappear, they are going to shadow you and try to pull you down. I had my share of the rough spots as I pushed through my journey to health and wellness, and I must tell you that the best way I discovered to get through them was to pray and ask God for strength and encouragement. He never failed me, I moved through many a tough area in the three years it took me to lose the weight I had to lose but when I called on the Lord, He did not disappoint. He is a very pleasant help in time of trouble and will see you through tough times if you give him the opportunity.

In the second year of my weight loss, I started to notice a couple of things. I knew they were there, but I never really got to see them. I used them every day, but the sight of them was hidden by parts of my anatomy and in the course of my lifetime as an obese man, I never realized how wonderful they were, how dependable and strong. One day I looked down and saw them and it was a delightful discovery, not only could I see my feet, but I was able to bend over and touch them, then sit on a chair or the edge of the bed and put my socks and shoes on all by myself without the help of an aide. This is something a lot of people take advantage of and unless your feet have been hiding behind a bump of fat for most of your life, you don't really see them as something special and worthy of such appreciation, but I will never forget the time when I was able to look down and see my feet, to actually be able to touch and dress them. It was a monumental moment.

In July of 2012 I declared my independence from fat and the tyranny it had made in my life, about a year and a half later I began to celebrate that independence. I will never forget the independence I felt when I was able to shower by myself, to be able to walk to the bathroom with no qualms or hesitation, no getting out of breath, no aches in my back or legs. I undressed myself, got into the tub needing no assistance, then dried off and dressed myself, it was quite an event.

I remember the cry of independence when I realized I did not need that giant truck any longer to get around. I sold my Sierra truck and was able to buy a Ford Taurus to drive around it. Not only was it a vivacious victory to go from a giant truck to a smaller car because I was slimming down, it was quite a triumph when I saw the difference in my gasoline bill for the month. I was saving a lot of money.

I heard the bells of independence when I went to the park, the mall, the store and festivals, too, now. I used to have to ride in my handicap scooter to enjoy being a spectator at these events, but now I could walk and enjoy sitting in a booth for a meal, experiencing a ride at a festival if I chose, pushing a cart around Walmart or the grocery store with no problem.

I enjoy Georgia's southern sporting events now, too. Football, baseball and basketball games are not a dream for me anymore, I don't have to wait to hear the stories about them from friends who were lucky enough to go to them, I'm lucky enough to make any sports game I choose to now. I love walking from the car through the crowd of fans into the stadium or arena, feeling the charge of excitement of being a Georgian in a state that takes its sports seriously.

And when it comes to celebrating independence, I have fireworks going off every time I am able to play sports with my brother. We go outside together and I don't have to sit in a chair to participate in a game of pitch and catch, I don't have to wait for him to get the ball for me if I don't catch it. We are equals out there on the ground of play, and that is one of the most magnificent feelings, to know that I was able to make the changes necessary that brought me to this place where I can experience the things I once thought were impossible.

If I want to go to a movie, I go with no trepidation or fear, I know now that I can fit into the seats and I don't have to worry about being embarrassed or fearful of breaking a chair.

I've been told that I am a lucky man to have had so much loving support during this time of distress and discovery. Not a lot of people are as lucky as I am, having a good family who loved me through it all and gave me the support I needed to get through the hard times and power through the changes that were necessary to take me from the pudgy little tadpole into a bouncing frog. I do not take them for granted, I am very grateful for every one of them and the help they have offered me. I know that without their help I would still be a prisoner today looking for hope and a solution to my growing problem.

A lot of people in my situation experience rejection, feelings of abandonment and despair. Many families grow frustrated and are worn down by the problems brought on by a morbidly obese loved one and I think in many situations it is easier to put them away or let them wallow in their condition behind a closed door to preserve any sort of peace and semblance of an ordinary life. I am very fortunate because I have such a super support system, my parents have been wonderful, my friends very supportive and my church family as well.

I can honestly say that I now feel normal, which is quite an understatement; after years of feeling like the elephant in the room, the fat guy, the one who couldn't fit in the booth or the seat, the one nobody wanted to sit next to on the plane or the bus. There have been many days when I would survey my life and be moved by disgust and have but one hope; to be normal. I wanted to know what it was like to sit, to stand, to walk, to run as a normal person, and not feel like I was being stared at, pointed to and laughed at. I recall saying this to someone once and being told that normal was just a setting on a washing machine, and that I should not put too much value into that mode of life, but in retrospect, I can tell you looking back to the man I was and seeing the man I am today, I have so many reasons to think that normal is much more than a washing machine setting.

I'm a single man with a hope of finding Mrs. Right and settling down to have a family someday. At one time, I had lost the hope for that kind of reality because I thought it was not fair to put a man of my size and health problems off on a woman, no matter how good and generous she was. Thanks to weight loss and finding a solution for my mental disability, that has changed and I now harbor the hope of settling down some day with the right woman to share my life with. I have no fears or trepidation in this area because I know that God will send me the woman of my dreams and together we will find all of the joy this life has to offer in the sense of happily ever after.

Finding my confidence was something that I doubted, even after losing a lot of weight I still doubted myself and fell short. It is often difficult for me to accept the reality of where I was and the man I have evolved into today. It has taken some getting used to and there are times when I feel displaced and uncomfortable, still plagued by the memories left in my charge from being over 500 pounds. I am able to go out now and engage in social activities and I feel as though I am not just existing now, I am living life to its fullest.

One of my greatest victories is my ministry, I no longer have to hold my sermons to a minute or two I can stand behind the pulpit and preach to my heart's content. The thing that I dreamed, the hope of fulfilling my calling from the Lord is now a reality and I am very happy about the work God has done and is doing in me. I told the Lord that if he would help me lose the weight, I would be obedient to him and do whatever he would have me do.

Today I am preaching more and more and seeing the physical changes, feeling the liberty it has given me, has had a positive effect on my personal growth and I have gained confidence to go out and go through whatever door opens to me.

Today I am very busy preaching and my zeal for God has made me stronger. I am blessed to move in the ministry today and I never forget the work God has done in me, and tell everyone I get the chance to meet that if God is for you, no one can keep you from experiencing the joy of victory, no matter who you are, where you come from, or how much you weigh.

When I think about the concepts of simply living and living life to its fullest, I realize that the man I was had no choice, he had to do whatever he could to simply survive and make it to the next day. That is not the case for me anymore. At birth I was given a gift of life, I did not always use that gift or honor it in the ways deemed necessary. I was not always wise in my choices and decisions, but today, I am living life to the fullest and enjoying every minute.

Chapter 10 - Paying It Forward

I remember sitting in a church service and hearing about how people don't need to go to a therapist or to see a psychiatrist. If we have the peace of God, we have all we need. We can go to God in prayer, we can get the counseling we need from Him and never have to worry about mental health. I believed that, I thought this was a get-out-of-jail-free card, or at least get out of the mental hospital free card, until I found myself in one wondering what sin I'd committed to land myself in there.

I felt weak, out of control, lost and full of self-animosity. I wanted a way out of my mental prison, the disorder I was suffering from and thought that if I prayed and prayed I would find one. I knew that prayer changed things and if I was a good enough Christian, I'd have faith, I'd have an answer and be able to live my life healed of any mental illness. I spent a lot of time praying and seeking God, but I still had the problem. It took me a long time to discover that the problem was not in me, in the illness I'd been afflicted with, the problem was in society and the beliefs I been tainted by.

It's been reported that three out of every four people with a mental illness experience stigma, that means that they feel marked with disgrace, a label that sets them apart from all of the 'normal' people. This is how stereotyping begins, people are set apart, put into specific groupings and given markers that make them different or special and then the negative attitudes and prejudices start piling up creating negative actions and discriminations.

Many times this stigma brings on feelings of shame, disgrace, and hopelessness. The affected person starts to be singled out and blamed for things that are not, in any way, his or her fault, but when something goes awry, they are the first to be blamed. This causes a high level of distress and soon the victims of such are being misrepresented by their peers and hiding from the help and resources that will bring them the help that they need. They hide their symptoms, disregard their medications refuse to go to doctor' s appointments—why? Because it makes them look like the crazies they are told about and they do not want to be lined up with such.

What I believe starts to happen here is that people begin to fear the label, and why wouldn't they?Mental Illness isn't exactly popular these days and there is no end to the name calling: loony, nuts, the weirdo, not playing with a full deck, the lights are on but there's no one at home, straight jacket wearers—the list continues. No one likes to be singled out especially if it means being put into a category that makes you out to be one of these.

Most people feel like being depressed is a sign of weakness and nobody is bragging about getting a high paying position in the work field because they suffer from depression, in fact most employers hesitate before hiring someone with a mental health illness. If you knew the guy running for president was subject to falling into a depression, would you give him your vote? That's usually one of the best vote killers in the United States. People just don't trust someone who is openly aware of their mental condition, be it depressed, bipolar, Obsessive Compulsive, Hyperactive, or just Schizoaffective. Is it any wonder that people with a mental health disability tend to do all they can to keep their condition a secret and wind up not getting the help they so need?

I spent a lot of time thinking about this after I was diagnosed with Schizoaffective Disorder, I felt all of these things and did not want people to put me down or into a class of nut jobs and whackos, I just wanted to ride the same train with everybody else so I did my best to keep my condition hush, hush and not say anything to anybody. That all changed once I started losing weight and lost the stigmas placed upon me for the disability or morbid obesity. As my confidence grew and I began to see myself in a different light, I realized that there was a lot of unfair treatment going on, not just for the obese, but for the mentally incapacitated.

I got so tired of the way mental health was being stigmatized, it was truly trying my nerves. Every time you turn on the news and hear about someone being hurt or murdered one of the first comments you hear is "Oh, that person must be nuts" or "he must be mentally ill!"

I have heard this all of my life and the truth is, when I realized I had a mental disorder, the first thing I thought of was that I had to be some kind of a nut and I was mentally ill! I didn't want that label, I didn't want people talking badly about me or putting me into that class of crazy so I fought my illness, tried to will it away, make it disappear.

It would not disappear, it would not fade no matter how I tried to make it go away. I put off treatment, tried to break out of the mental health hospital even refused to go for my follow up visits and wound up lying to the doctor because I was afraid of being stigmatized and I had every right to feel this way, society does not make it easy on the mentally handicapped.

I finally got tired of feeling this way and came to the realization that not everyone who did horrible things was just plain old crazy, sometimes people are just evil and they do evil things.

I thought things would be different in my faith community and I would find solace there, but the truth is the Christians who say you can't be depressed and know Christ are the same ones who point their fingers at those with mental handicaps and call them crazy and just not right with God. No one is exempt from a mental health disorder, just like no one is exempt from physical disorders. Just because you have diabetes doesn't mean you can't believe in God, the same goes for the Mental Health Illness victim, just because you have a mental health disorder, does not make you weak, weary in faith and incapable of believing God to work in your life.

I'm a simple man, but as I grew stronger and more self-assured, I began to realize that I could do something about this to make a difference. I knew it would not be easy, but I wanted to do something to help educate people and to get rid of the stigmas crippling society and their opinions of the mentally disabled. I decided to start a non-profit organization that would do just that, in 2005 I started pulling out the stops and looking for a way to make a difference. I called it "Recovery in Progress", because no one working on a disability can snap their fingers and find an instant cure, it is indeed, a process, and recovery is a progressive thing.

I don't have an office, I work at my computer using the internet as a window to reach as many people as possible to spread my cause. I do not have a staff of steady volunteers but when I work on events and fund raisers, I do find people to help me with that. The steady focus and thrust for my work is to educate the public on the actual facts about those living with a mental health diagnosis; I am a man who has a mental health diagnosis so I use my own personal experiences as a resource for what I am doing.

I started out small but as I go along, I am finding that doors are opening to me to work in a dynamic function to help not only dissolve the misconceptions put into place by people who don't truly understand what a mental handicap entails, but I am able to work hands on with those affected by a mental illness.

May is Mental Health Awareness Month and I think it is only fitting for me to do an annual mental health awareness night that incorporates fun recreational events, good music along with local celebrities on hand to meet and greet people in support of our cause. It is an event we have held for a few years now and every year it seems to get better and better. Every year we have a theme for the event, "Stamping Out Stigma", "Recovery In Progress", "Too Fit to Quit", "Staying Serene in 2014", and this year we are under the banner of "A Night of Hope".

I am currently working with some good people who want to help me with spreading the work about "Recovery in Progress", creating a website, a Facebook Page and an email newsletter. I believe that this is a remarkable opportunity for me to get the word out about this very important cause and I am taking full advantage of it.

I am a man with a vision; Recovery in Progress is an organization I would like to take to a national level, doing events not just in southern Georgia but all over this great nation of ours.

I would like to do work like I see being done by the National Alliance for the Mentally Ill (NAMI) and Depression and Bipolar Support Alliance (DBSA).

I have been blessed with volunteers who carry the vision of Recovery in Progress. Three of those volunteers are my good friends and biggest supporters, Billy Johnson, Kathy Durden, and David Crooke. Kathy Durden and David Cooke run a local business Care Partners of Georgia that work with Children with Behavioral Health Progress and developmental disabilities. They always help me out each year with providing food for the attendees at the event every year. I could not have such a successful event annually if it was not for my awesome volunteers. Whatever the job, setting up chairs and booths, distributing tickets, arranging door prizes and drawings, setting up musical entertainment, I have a list of people who are there every year to help make our event a success.

When I think about all that has occurred in my life with my weight problems, my dependency on food, and the mental health condition I have, Schizoaffective Disorder, I find myself feeling more and more blessed to be able to walk through my issues and discover the strength to not just deal with them, but to overcome them.

It is not an easy thing to live with an emotional illness, many times people have something going on and are too afraid to face the facts, too afraid to want to find the help they need to begin the healing so that they, too, can experience a recovery in progress. Usually hurt feelings are pushed aside, dysfunctional reactions are passed off as the norm or just what's average for me and seeking professional help is not often an option or a path taken.

My disability was not one that could be hidden, I could not pretend I was not over 300 pounds overweight. I could not ignore the physical limitations I was experiencing or the health problems that ensued as a result of it. I had to face my dilemma and hope for a solution. I had to find the strength from within myself and apply my faith in God knowing that He was able to do great things and take over where my strength lacked. I am not a superman in any way, form or fashion, I know my limits, my problems, my weaknesses; but I am also aware of my strengths: strength to move forward, strength to face many obstacles and against all odds make a way to find peace and happiness for myself.

What I have done is nothing unusual or out of the ordinary, many people experience obesity, many fall victim to the trials of life and use food for more than the fuel it was designed to be for our bodies. I have seen so many people with incredible stories, stories of hope, redemption and atonement. I get excited every time I see someone overcoming addictions, to food or otherwise, and walking a journey that takes them from frustration, fed up with life the way it was and to contentment, heightened self-esteem and bliss. I walked that path, I experienced that bliss and now I want to share it with others.

When I see a person struggling with a mental health disorder, I find myself wanting to help them, to reach out to them and give them a helping hand, to not just walk one mile with them, but to make the journey of the second mile as well. I feel as though I have been given a gift and I know God has appointed me to spread this truth: no matter what has fallen on you, no matter what your situation, you can find a way to get out and live a happy, healthy life.

Chapter 11 - Many Thanks

Back in the day, when I was not fortunate enough to buy a gym membership, I was given a gift. It came from a woman who was very encouraging and never stopped believing in me, even when I had serious doubts about myself. Her name was Carolyn Braswell, she owned and operated CPR Fitness, and this a fitness center, and she made me an offer to come and workout whenever I wanted to at no charge. I am so grateful for her generosity and giving spirit, she truly helped make the difference I was needing.

There were many who I call angels who have helped me along my way, one I call a God-send, Mr. Don Wages, who was my physical therapist at the Nursing Home. This man was always there for me, he understood my position and mindset even when I did not get it myself. He motivated me, pushed me when I was in a stall, when I didn't think I could move forward he had a way of opening a door and pushing me through it in spite of the fact that I felt like I was incapable of walking. He took a vested interest in my life; after I was released from the nursing home, Don continued to call me and motivated me to move and progress to meet my goals. I am forever grateful.

Working out as man over 500 pounds is no picnic, it was not something I wanted to do or thought physically possible, but that changed when I met Robert Allen, a trainer at CPR Fitness. I was of the opinion that there were certain body parts that were glued in place and impossible to work, but thanks to Mr. Robert, I learned how to move and work out correctly so that it would benefit my physical condition. He would work with me at the gym and give me printouts to help me along my fitness journey and never gave up on me. He was without a doubt another shining star, one who I could not have found my way to health and happiness without.

Live Healthy M.D., in Augusta, Georgia, is where my medical adventure began. It started with my surgeon, Dr. Darren Glass, who was a magnificent man of medicine and started me on my journey to health.

Another doctor at Live Healthy M.D., Dr. Edward Boland, was my medical weight loss doctor who was given the task of helping me lose 100 pounds prior to surgery. When I first met him, I was at my highest weight, he was tenacious in spite of my up and down, yo-yo dieting process. He did some research and discovered a program called the Duke Diet.

He knew this would work for me because I liked lots of meat and would snack a lot, so as long as I followed this diet of high protein offerings, I could lose the weight. He was correct and helped me to lose 100 pounds.

Trish Fine and Bryn Hamilton are nutritionists/dietitians at Live Healthy M.D., and they taught me all about eating. When to eat, what to eat, how much to eat, what not to eat, what time to eat--all of my eating questions and problems were answered by these two wonderful ladies and they were most gracious in their work with me and taught me so much about nutrition.

I am so grateful to the entire staff at Live Healthy M.D., the nurses, the office staff and the techs were all so helpful and kind to me throughout my entire weight loss journey and I want them all to know how much I appreciate everything they have done for me.

Dr. Troy Austin, from Southeastern Aesthetic Surgery in Evans, Georgia, is the surgeon who did my tummy tuck. Being such a large man has a tendency to rob you of many things; self-assurance, confidence, the ability to love yourself. Working with the professionals at Dr. Austin's office, I was able to come to grips with the man I actually am and thanks to their generosity, courtesy and helpful support, I was able to be introduced to the man I have always known I could be, from the inside out.

The staff of Uni Post-Acute Care, formerly known as Heritage Health Care, in Swainsboro, Georgia, the nursing home I was in, deserves a heartfelt thanks for all of their care and helpful support during my stay there. They were very well-informed and took care of me and my special needs in a most professional and considerate way and I will always be indebted to them for their help.

I want to give special consideration to the office of Dr. James Ray, my medical doctor, and his staff for all that they have done for me in my journey. Carrie Ray, a Physician's Assistant, was most gracious and helpful to me during this time.

Had it not been for her advice and direction, I would not have begun my trek to health. She was the one who pointed me to the path of weight loss surgery and let me know that there were answers to my questions and hope for my transformation.

Brenda Thompson has been a constant companion throughout my expedition to wellness, she has been with me from East Georgia Health Care to Dr. Ray's office and even when I was seeing Carrie Ray, Brenda would pop in from time to time to see how I was doing. Her undying support and continual care is what sets her aside from most medical professionals today and I appreciate her so much.

No thanksgiving offering on my part would be complete without my saying thanks and paying tribute to my best friend, Ben Braswell. Ben has always been there for me, from our childhood when we played baseball together to our adult years when life got tough and bumpy, I always knew that I could depend on Ben. He has been my constant friend and confidant, offering me support in the tough times, dispensing advice when I needed it and just holding me up when I felt like I could not stand on my own. Friendships are a gift of God and I am forever grateful for this treasure the Lord has bestowed upon me.

Southside Baptist Church is a fellowship of believers who take the idea of church family seriously, they are without a doubt, an extended part of my family and have always treated me as such. Their undying support, constant companionship and holding me up in prayer 24 hours a day seven days a week is something I just could not have made it without and for that I am blessed and grateful.

I want to pay particular attention to my former pastor, Pastor Earl Warnock, who has retired but is now named Pastor Emeritus, in my church, giving him a life time honorary pastorship at Southside Baptist Church. Where do I begin and how can I say thank you to such a man of faith, honor, integrity and benevolence? He was there for me in times of hurt and seasons of calamity; walking me through the path God put before me, offering me direction and guidance. He was also there when I found my faith and confidence and came to a joyous victory and helped me celebrate my renovation. Without a doubt, this man was one of my biggest super supporters and I am eternally thankful to him and the work he has done on this planet and in my life.

My current pastor is Chad Kennison, who I have known for over three years now. In this short time he has shown himself to be a true man of God, compassionate and full of Godly wisdom. I want to thank him for helping me through this time and always being there to pray for me and guide me through times of strife and despair and for leading me to a joyous conclusion.

Pastor Jayson Keefer, a former pastor from New Beginnings Baptist Church, deserves mention, because he went above and beyond the call of duty and truly walked the second mile with me in my quest for health. Pastor Keefer would come out to my house every morning at seven or eight o'clock to make sure I was exercising and moving forward in my weight loss program. You won't find a lot of people with that kind of dedication, and this meant an awful lot to me and I am most grateful.

Last and not least, my thanks goes to my family. They have always supported me, held me up, pushed me forward, slapped my hand, continued to speak words of love and sustenance into me and never let me fall without rushing to my side to help me get back on my feet, physically as well as emotionally.

They have prayed with me, cried with me, celebrated with me and they are the inspiration that has been my one true constant throughout this entire process. I am a blessed man, half the size I used to be, but this journey has done a work on me giving me a double portion of love, purpose and intent that I will use wisely as I move forward into my future.

Chapter 12 - Super Supporters

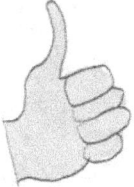

Oh what a journey, I've had highs and lows, fast and slows but I made it and I am a happy and healthy man today thanks to the Grace of God and I got by with a lot of help from my friends. This chapter is dedicated to them, my super supporters who were there for me through thick and thin.

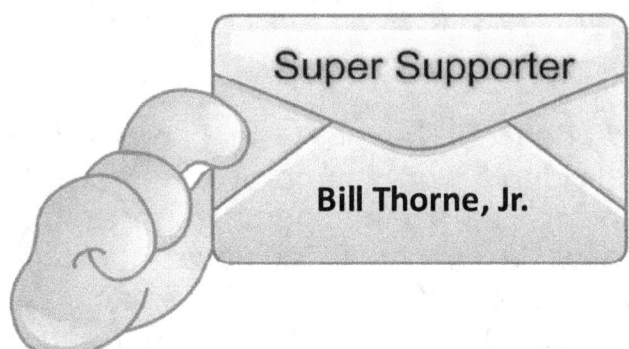

Super Supporter

Bill Thorne, Jr.

As a long-time friend of Danny's, since we were teenagers, I have witnessed his many struggles with obesity and both the physical, emotional, and psychological impact this has had on his life.

For many years Danny was over 500 pounds, making it almost impossible to function in a normal capacity. I knew Danny well enough to know that he would be one of those dedicated and few people who would conquer this and, therefore, his amazing transformation came as no surprise to me.

This amazing process in seeing him go from over 500 pounds to 225 pounds in what seemed to be a very short time has been phenomenal and inspirational to a lot of people. I know that Danny's dedication coupled with his trust in God to help him accomplish this feat has gotten him to this point.

We are all in awe of Danny and know that anyone who reads his story will be inspired as well.

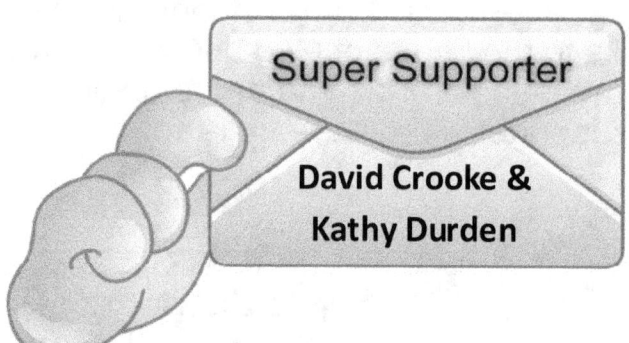

Super Supporter

David Crooke &
Kathy Durden

SAMSHA defines Recovery as a process of change whereby individuals work to improve their own health and wellness and to live a meaningful life in a community of their choice while striving to achieve their full potential. This definition exemplifies Danny Coleman. We had the privilege to meet Danny Coleman 10 years ago as a part of his recovery journey. Danny had a vision to sponsor a Mental Health Awareness Day in Swainsboro, Georgia, which is a rural county that has a population of approximately 5000 residents. He reached out to a friend of esteemed colleague, Larry Fricks and ours. Larry is internationally known for his work designing and crafting the first Medicaid-billable Certified Peer Specialist program in the United States during his nearly 13 years as director of Georgia's Office of Consumer Relations and Recovery in the Division of Mental Health, Developmental Disabilities and Addictive Diseases. He is a founder of Georgia's Peer Specialist Training and Certification; and a founder of the Georgia Peer Support Institute. He served on the Planning Board for the 1999 Surgeon General's Report on Mental Health, and currently serves on the Board of Directors of Mental Health America (MHA, formerly the National Mental Health Association). He also sits on the Carter Center's Advisory Board for the Rosalynn Carter Fellowships for Mental Health Journalism. Larry called us and said, I have a friend that wants to plan a mental health awareness night, and can you guys support him. We said absolutely. Larry shared how impressed he was that this young man invested his time, energy and effort to research mental health community awareness activities on the internet and through that process had discovered Larry's contact information. Danny "sold" Larry on his dream and Larry embraced this dream and wanted to support him. This process defines "peer support" at its best. Larry also advocated and linked him to others to foster relationships and establish needed community supports to promote Danny's hopes and dreams. When we met Danny, he already had his vision firmly mapped out. Danny had thoroughly mapped this event out from A-Z, from his Recovery theme, to flyers, to T-Shirts, to motivational speakers, to inviting local state Governmental officials, to regional entertainers, he had covered all of his bases. Basically, Danny just needed our organization to be a sponsor for refreshments. That would be easy for us to do. Although both of us have supported the Georgia Mental Health Consumer Network and it's Peer Support Program, and are very versed in the concept of recovery and person center planning, the idea of being a partner and not an expert in the field of behavioral health services, our relationship with Danny over the last 10 years have solidified our belief that RECOVERY is possible by following certain principles. Danny has taught us more regarding these principles through his lived experience then any textbook or college degree ever could. As the 10 years passed, Danny's vision evolved and expanded. The event has become an annual tradition in small town America. He has shown dedication in his commitment to plan and host this event. The event has become a living testimony of Danny's perseverance, and his unshakable faith, and the power of his optimism and his belief in hope.

This event has also become a testimony of how Danny uses his strengths, abilities and talents to obtain his life goals. Mental Health consumers have for too long only been viewed by the community and the uninformed professionals that serve them through the lens of their diagnosis and the stigma that has been attached to their illness. This stigma, all too often has created multiple barriers that cause the person with mental illness to be viewed using terms like weaknesses and deficits. Danny posses enumerable skills and talents and this event has fostered them immensely. Danny is a marvelous broker and coordinator of community resources. He possesses an amazing aptitude for salesmanship and has learned the skill that would make many skilled salesmen green with envy, "Don't let the first block stop you". This event has become a catalyst of growth for his public speaking skills. Danny has become a confident Emcee of this event and has played host to SEC football players, State Senators, Judges, Ministers, Mental Health Professionals, Peers and the general public alike. Danny meets all with his relaxed, laid-back manner that readily sets people at ease and makes this occasion a success year after year. However, not only have we had the privilege to see the event grow we have seen Danny reach many goals he set for himself.

As he began his journey of mental health wellness, he also began to transform physically before our eyes. Danny has lost over 300 lbs. He has demonstrated holistic wellness through his mental, physical, and spiritual commitments that are steadfast in his daily living. He has presented at the Georgia Mental Health Conference in St. Simons, Georgia on how to plan and organize a Mental Health Awareness Day in your own hometown. He has recently attended the Peer Support Certification Program and passed the written and oral exams and has now become a Certified Peer Specialist.

The best way to describe the accomplishments of Danny's journey is actually use the SAMSHA principles of recovery and present how he has demonstrated each of these principles in his continued journey.

Person-driven--Danny possesses the skills and abilities to express his life goals and preferences. He has the uncanny strength to partner with multiple community and family resources to attain these goals.

Occurs via many pathways--Danny's recovery path includes traditional Mental Health services, support groups such as weight watchers, peer support, his church, community supports and the support of his family.

Is holistic; this has been one of the hallmarks of his recovery. Danny has developed an awareness of the importance of holistic and integrated recovery that incorporates the mind, body and spirit. Danny's religious and spiritual beliefs have been a foundational strength and natural support for his recovery efforts.

Is supported by peers; Danny's growth and recovery has incorporated the resources of the local state and regional recovering community. Danny uses social media to reach out to peers across the state. By sharing his lived experience, Danny has enriched our local community and has demonstrated to them that people with mental illness can thrive.

Is supported through relationships; Danny's ability to bring diverse people together has become an amazing asset for the recovery movement. Some of the supported relationships we have seen Danny cultivate include, NAMI, Georgia Mental Health Consumer Network, University of Georgia Football Program, Swainsboro Jaycees, Swainsboro Fire Department, Stitch in Print, (donates T-Shirts each year) Emanuel County Art Center, Sam's Drive-In Band, Southside Baptist Church and various Church choirs and quartets. Many of the local business donate door prizes for the event.

Is culturally-based and influenced; the attendance of the event reflects the diversity of our community. Danny demonstrates sensitivity to the diverse needs of our community through his speaker selection.

Is supported by addressing trauma; Speakers share their lived experience that includes their personal stories of trauma.

Involves individual, family, and community strengths and responsibility; we have discussed the strengths of Danny and the community members in previous examples. We want to acknowledge and highlight the vast amount of support that Danny's family has demonstrated during the past ten years. Danny's family exhibits positive regard and support toward his recovery.

They have a strong commitment and dedication in supporting his dreams of expanding his program known as Recovery in Progress. We have witnessed their own growth in understanding recovery and mental illness.

Is based on respect; Danny demonstrates a deep respect, admiration for the cause of battling stigma, educating others regarding mental illness and recovery. He highlights other's qualities and is dedicated to continue a public forum for other's to share their story in their own words emerges from hope. Danny holds on, perseveres, and believes in a better tomorrow.

We are both proud and honored that Danny allowed us to share a part of his journey and we continue to support his continue journey. We have no doubt that he is just beginning many accomplishments to come.

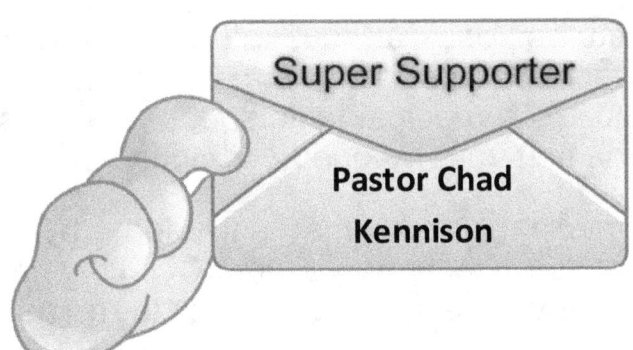

Super Supporter

Pastor Chad Kennison

I have known Danny for a little over 3 years now. I remember the first time I met Danny, he weighed over five hundred pounds. I remember that it seemed like it was a struggle just to move around. I remember when he first started talking about having surgery, and there was a certain amount of weight to lose. I remember the determination he had! This seems to mark the attitude that Danny has had throughout his remarkable journey.

After the surgery Danny has been able to maintain his determination, and has stayed the course. Now I see Danny as a vibrant individual with a spring in his step, and a determination to help others that face similar problems. Danny is a very talented individual with pen and words, and it comes out every time he writes. Danny has also been a source of encouragement to our church family, and is always ready to give a testimony of his success, and give God all the glory for it.

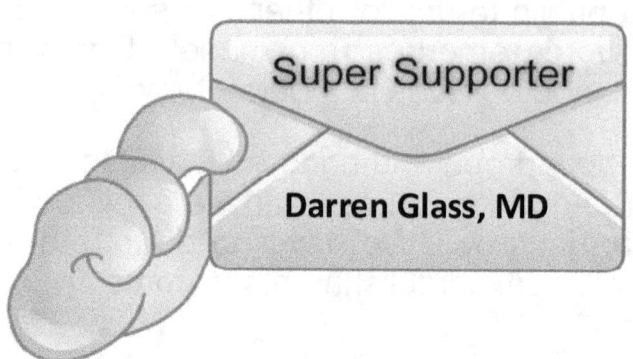

Well, pictures speak a thousand words, and looking at your pictures from the time I met you in 11 to now, enough said. The medical facts speak for themselves as well. When I met you weighed 444 pounds.

Your medical problems included hypertension, diabetes, congestive heart failure, COPD, and asthma. You took twelve daily medications to manage these problems.

You came with your mother, not only because she is a wonderful lady who cares about you, but because you needed her to take care of you.

Look at you now.   One gastric bypass, an appendectomy, and a paniculectomy later, you are confident, independent and healthy. Your weight is stable in the 220s. Although still on a few medications for blood pressure, lungs, and mood, you are much healthier than you were and please imagine (not for too long) what life would be like now, a few years older, at 444 pounds or worse. You are active in your community, church and school, and have a bright future ahead of you.

I want to praise you, encourage you and warn you. Look where you came from, look where you are now, and look ahead to where God is leading you. From a weight loss perspective, remember these rules: one cup meals, three meals a day; solid meaty foods, mostly meat, a little vegetables, minimal snacking and exercise. Lt these four simple principles guide you through a healthy lifestyle that will last a lifetime.

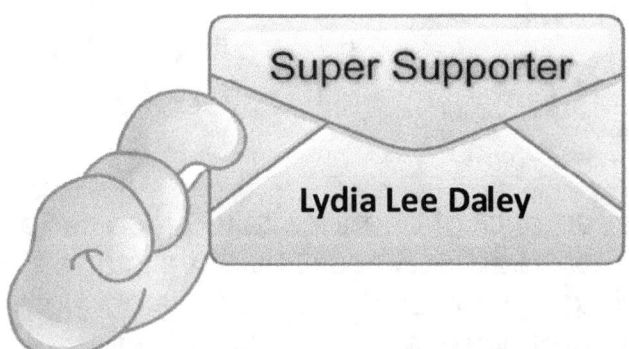

Super Supporter

Lydia Lee Daley

I have known Danny Coleman, as his treating physician, for over 10 years. He initially was attending a day program at our facility where patients go to learn skills to manage their mental illness. Danny was always friendly and outgoing and made friends easily. He wanted to help people early on but he was hampered due to health issues

I have seen Danny transform from a slightly shy and insecure person to one who knows what he wants and goes after it. He has more confidence and he has become a champion for mental health awareness. I think Danny is just getting started.

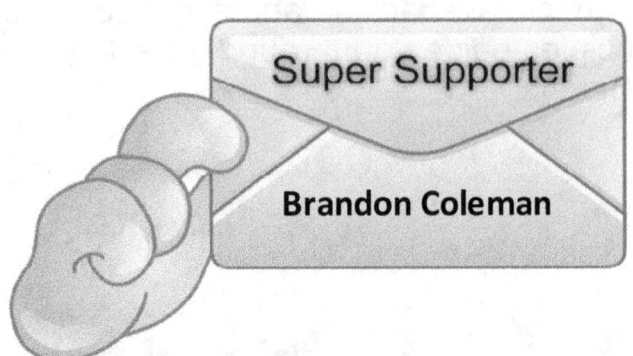

Super Supporter

Brandon Coleman

I have seen a lot of changes take place in you over the last couple of years. Since you have started losing the weight through your diet and the weight loss surgery, everything about you has seemed to change.

You have become much more energetic, you actually do a lot of your own stuff now, and you seem to feel better about yourself. You have made me proud and you are a huge inspiration to not only us as your family, but also to everyone around you. People that hear your story and all the problems that you have overcome cannot help but to be inspired to be a better person. Whether that's pushing them to do something about their weight or any other facet of life, your story shows them that if they really try hard to do something, they can do it.

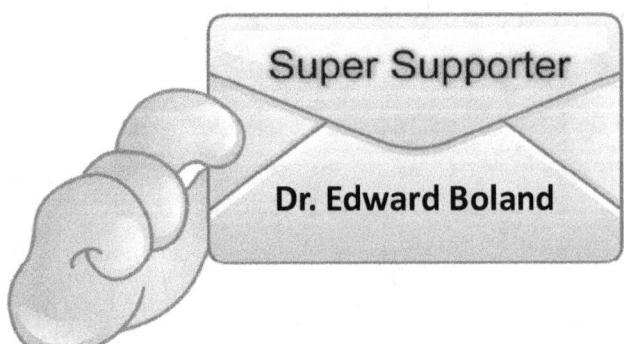

Super Supporter

Dr. Edward Boland

It's been said that "obesity is a super highway with lots of on-ramps." Danny recognized this and was very smart to use all of his available resources to fight against the many "on-ramps" that would get in his way. It was impressive to me that a member (or two) from Danny's family came with him to each visit. So much information is exchanged in such a short time at patient appointments, that it's very important to take notes and have supporters that can help recall exactly what the doctor said. When new questions arose between visits, Danny or his family would contact the office for clarification, so no time was wasted.

When it comes to weight loss, many people automatically think of diet and exercise. Unfortunately, they usually don't know how and are stuck using whatever the latest TV gimmick suggests. Danny got the support of his family and community to help him maintain a diet that was different from anything most of them had ever tried before. He was open to trying medications beyond the typically well-known "diet pills." Most importantly, Danny was open to the most overlooked (and most important) parts of weight loss, behavior modification. By having his family, friends, and church community understand his goals and not "sabotage" his efforts with inappropriate offers of foods, Danny was able to make dramatic changes in a very short period of time.

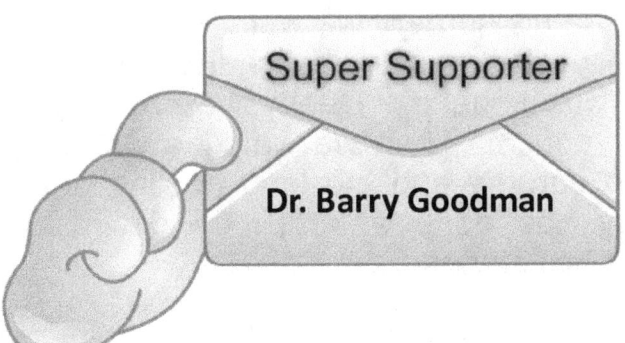

Six years ago I met Danny Coleman while preaching a Revival in his home church. He was a large man and had a huge appetite for the Word of God. The next year when

I returned for another meeting Danny had drastically changed physically but had retained his wonderful sweet spirit and desire to please God. Danny Coleman had a severe challenge but chose to depend on an Omnipotent God to see him through the obstacles that faced him. He is an inspiration and example of what one can do through the power of our Lord Jesus Christ. My life and ministry has been enriched by my acquaintance with Danny Coleman.

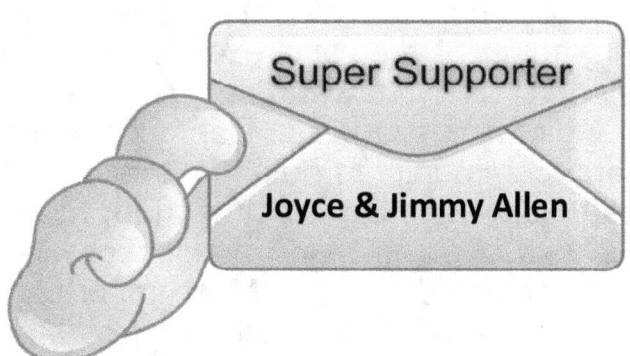

Super Supporter

Joyce & Jimmy Allen

It has been a joy to know and fellowship with Danny Coleman Jr. When Danny first came to our church he was very quiet, kind, and polite. When we met Danny he was already on his journey of success and it was so much fun to watch him as he journeyed down his road. We prayed for him, as we know what a struggle it is to diet, then when he his surgery we watched the pounds just fall off. Some of the men at the church were beginning to suck their gut in haha. Danny was making them think about their pouch. Then we watched Danny go through the second surgery and the long healing process. Now that Danny has gone a long way down that road to success he just shines.

He is so active in church and community events. He still remains kinda quiet, kind, and polite but he is not sitting still. He goes, goes, and goes. Also, I have noticed that Danny is a very organized person. He does a Mental Health Awareness Event every year and for the past 3 years he has shared with me what all he is doing. I am impressed. Many people I know can take lessons from him. I don't think Danny has completed his journey to success, he is just gonna take another road for a different destination. He hasn't finished yet--just wait and see!

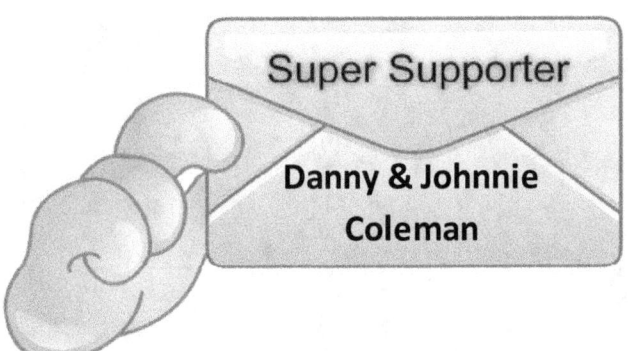

Letter from Danny Ray Coleman, Sr. and Johnnie Faye Coleman; Danny, Jr.'s Parents:

It has been an experience of joy, heartache, and happiness being Danny's parents. We have watched him overcome all the tough times in his life. From being over 500 lbs to less than 250; from being an honor roll student through school to having a mental breakdown and going through some rough times; from being lost in a world of sin to being called by the Lord to serve Him at a young age and has never stopped even through his tough times. Oh what memories come to mind, a little boy with a western outfit, wrestling outfit, baseball and football player, being in a mental hospital, being confined to home because of weight, all kinds of health problems, having to move slow when we did go somewhere so he could keep up, to not being able to keep up with him now. I remember watching his mother cry in worry, to being over ran with joy at the results of his hard work. He truly named this book correctly "Half the Man I used to be with twice the heart!" Danny's life is all about helping others today, and he does it well. So many people has been inspired by his journey, and I think that he has only just begun. To see him today as a man who cares for others including his little brother. Seeing his concern about other's needs really makes me see what love really is. God is good, and we as a family are greatly blessed!

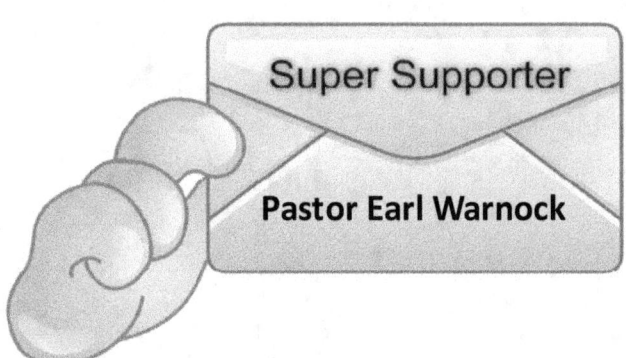

Super Supporter

Pastor Earl Warnock

I got to know Danny about four years ago. Danny was a big fellow, weighing over 500 pounds. Danny could not do hardly anything for himself. His family had to dress him. He could not sit in an ordinary chair.

Most times, Danny had to lay down. His family would get him dressed, and carry him to church, where he desired to go. Danny began to have a real desire to be like other young men, and to be able to do things for himself and for others. Danny began to follow Doctor's advice, to lose weight. I have seen Danny sit at the table, while others were eating all the tasty foods, but Danny took control of his life, and started losing weight. He did not let his appetite for food, control his desire for a healthy body. This young man found a way to discipline himself in so many ways. He got into an exercise program. If there has ever been a young fellow that could be an example setter, for others to follow in so many different ways, Danny Coleman, Jr. is the man. I truly admire him for the way he has disciplined himself.

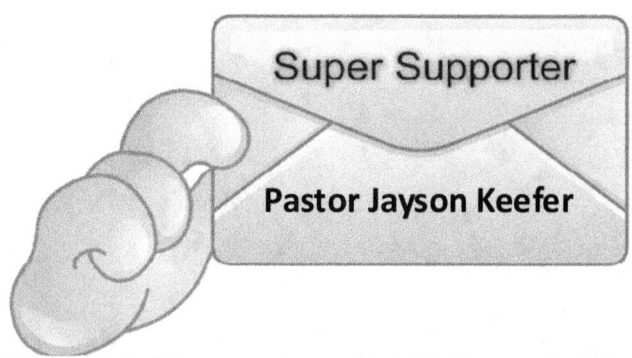

Super Supporter

Pastor Jayson Keefer

I met Danny in the spring of 2009, and right away the one thing I knew was he wanted to make a difference. His determination and faithfulness has made an impact on his family as well as others. With such a passionate heart it has been no wonder that Danny's obstacles could not hold him back.

It seems there have been times where Danny felt as though he had little or no purpose, and would surely give up. I remember once trying to help him by walking with him each day, and when I would leave I thought for sure he had given up all together. Sooner or later he would always come back around, refusing defeat.

I know of people today whose lives are at a standstill because they cannot get past some of the same problems Danny has faced. His faith in Christ has been the determining factor in his success. Persevering through the hard times has left a testimony that is sure to help others in the years to come.

I look forward to seeing how God will continue to use this man whose heart has been yielded to the leading of his master, Jesus Christ.

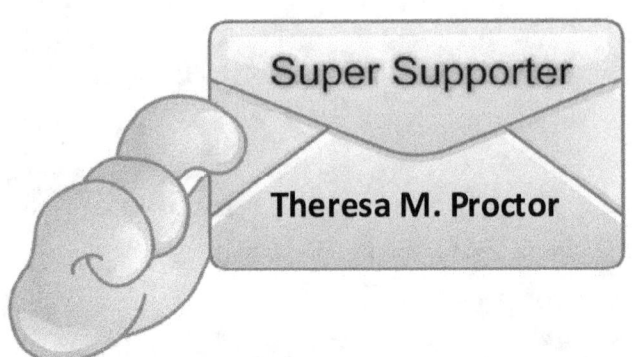

Super Supporter

Theresa M. Proctor

As a Weight Watchers leader I have the privilege of guiding members toward making choices that will lead them to living a healthy lifestyle. This requires a lot of change which can be difficult. Oftentimes these changes become overwhelming and members will struggle and some give up. Learning to be patient and to make small changes is what will lead to a member's true success. Finding out that success is not measured by that number on the scale alone but by all of the many 'mini' changes is what it is all about. I am so thankful to have been a small part of Danny's journey.

He is one of those members that will forever be an inspiration and source of motivation to me and countless others. When I first met him, he was quiet, nervous and overwhelmed with the task ahead. I also saw, however, a look of determination in his eyes and I knew he had what it took to persevere. He just had to learn to believe it.

Each week at our meetings, it is my goal to guide members toward making small, realistic goals. Danny, although faced with many obstacles, took on each weekly challenge with vigor. Watching him change was absolutely amazing. One week we discussed the importance of exercise and the role it plays in living a healthy lifestyle. I challenged the members that week to set a small goal regarding activity. Danny confessed to me that he had been given a treadmill and it had been on his porch for nearly a year, untouched. I asked him to set his goal for that week to move the treadmill into the house. 'You don't even have to turn it on!' I told him. 'We'll work on that next week.'

Over the course of time, he went from barely being able to walk on that treadmill to becoming a member of a gym with a personal trainer! His perseverance and determination transformed him from that nervous, overwhelmed young man into a confident inspiration to many others. He learned that making small changes leads to huge results on and off that scale. He passed that knowledge onto others who were struggling each week, becoming a motivating force. He has completely changed his relationship with food and continues to practice healthy habits.

He really gets it. He knows that the number on the scale is not the only way to measure his success. I have been privileged to have half the opportunity to watch him change into a confident, healthy young man.

Danny, I am honored to have been a part of your journey. I am so proud of you and what you have achieved. I have all the confidence that you will continue to persevere and become very successful. I look forward to sharing in more of those successes! Thank you for allowing me to be a part of your amazing accomplishments.

Sincerely,

Theresa M. Proctor

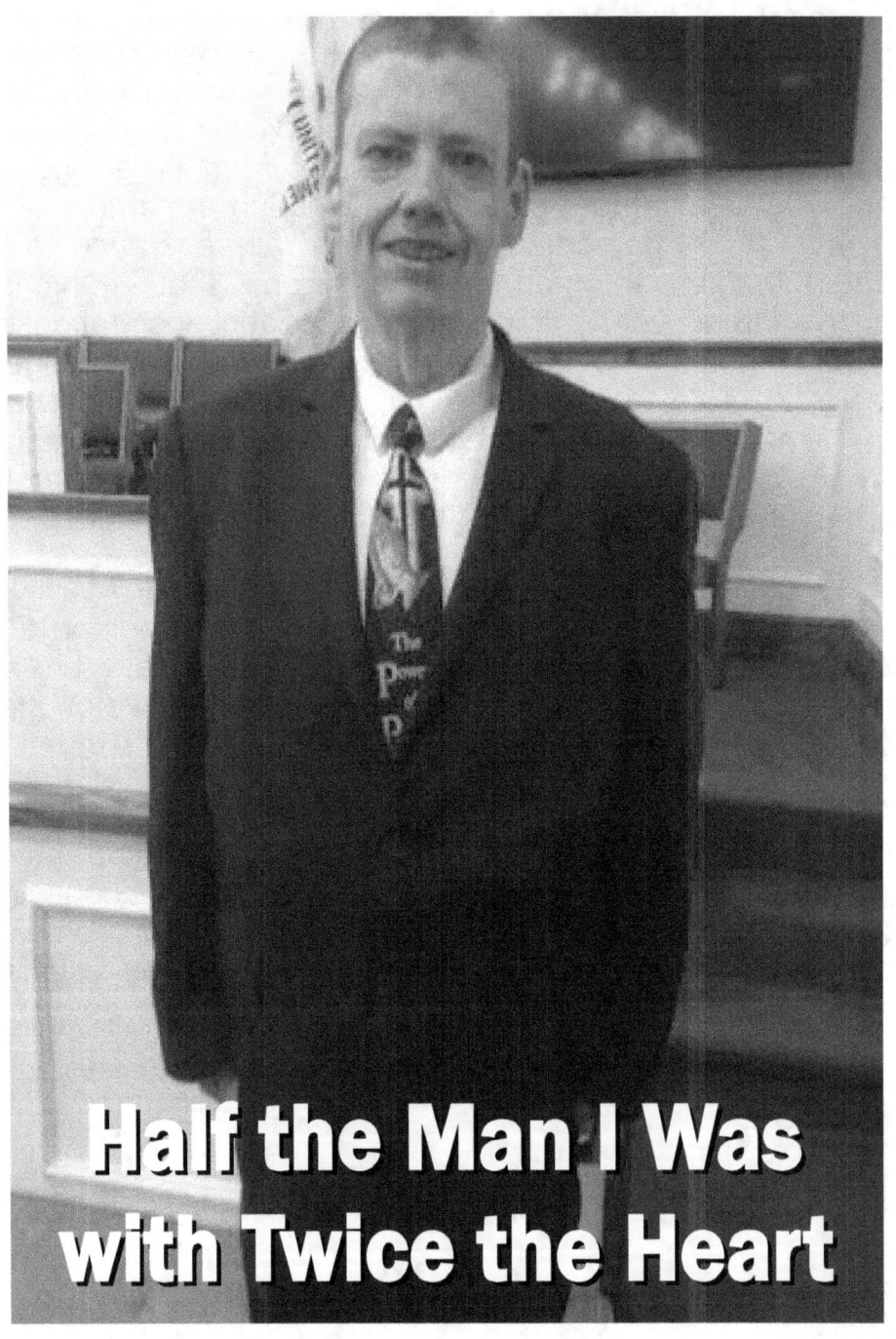

Half the Man I Was with Twice the Heart

www.ingramcontent.com/pod-product-compliance
Lightning Source LLC
Chambersburg PA
CBHW071211280526
45787CB00002B/642